BLACKWELL

UNDERGROUND CLINICAL VIGNETTES

MICROBIOLOGY II: BACTERIOLOGY, 4E

BLACKWELL

UNDERGROUND CLINICAL VIGNETTES

MICROBIOLOGY II: BACTERIOLOGY

VIKAS BHUSHAN, MD
Series Editor
University of California, San Francisco, Class of 1991
Diagnostic Radiologist

VISHAL PALL, MD MPH
Series Editor
Internist and Preventive Medicine Specialist
Government Medical College, Chandigarh – Panjab University – India, Class of 1997
Graduate School of Biomedical Sciences at UTMB Galveston, MPH, Class of 2004

TAO LE, MD
University of California, San Francisco, Class of 1996

KAUSHIK MUKHERJEE
David Geffen School of Medicine at UCLA, Class of 2005

SAMEER SHETH, PhD
David Geffen School of Medicine at UCLA, Class of 2005

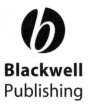

Blackwell
Publishing

© 2005 by Blackwell Publishing

Blackwell Publishing, Inc., 350 Main Street, Malden, Massachusetts 02148-5018, USA
Blackwell Publishing Ltd, 9600 Garsington Road, Oxford OX4 2DQ, UK
Blackwell Publishing Asia Pty Ltd, 550 Swanston Street, Carlton, Victoria 3053, Australia

05 06 07 08 5 4 3 2 1

ISBN-13: 978-1-4051-0413-5
ISBN-10: 1-4051-0413-9

Library of Congress Cataloging-in-Publication Data

Microbiology. Bacteriology / Vikas Bhushan . . . [et al.].— 4th ed.
    p. ; cm. — (Blackwell underground clinical vignettes)
  Rev. ed. of: Microbiology, v. 3 / Vikas Bhushan. 3rd ed. c2002.
  ISBN-13: 978-1-4051-0413-5 (pbk. : alk. paper)
  ISBN-10: 1-4051-0413-9 (pbk. : alk. paper) 1. Medical bacteriology—Case studies.
  2. Physicians—Licenses—United States—Examinations—Study guides.
  [DNLM: 1. Bacterial Infections—Case Reports. 2. Bacterial Infections—Problems and
Exercises. 3. Bacteriology—Case Reports. 4. Bacteriology—Problems and Exercises. 5. Parasitic
Diseases—Case Reports. 6. Parasitic Diseases—Problems and Exercises. WC 18.2 B131 2005]
  I. Bhushan, Vikas. II. Bhushan, Vikas. Microbiology. III. Series: Blackwell's underground clinical
vignettes.

  QR46.B23 2005
  616.9'201'076—dc22

                                                                                            2005003545

A catalogue record for this title is available from the British Library

Acquisitions: Nancy Anastasi Duffy
Development / Production: Jennifer Kowalewski
Cover and Interior design: Leslie Haimes
Typesetter: Graphicraft in Quarry Bay, Hong Kong
Printed and bound by Capital City Press in Berlin, VT

For further information on Blackwell Publishing, visit our website:
www.blackwellmedstudent.com

NOTICE

The indications and dosages of all drugs in this book have been recommended in the medical literature and conform to the practices of the general community. The medications described do not necessarily have specific approval by the Food and Drug Administration for use in the diseases and dosages for which they are recommended. The package insert for each drug should be consulted for use and dosage as approved by the FDA. Because standards for usage change, it is advisable to keep abreast of revised recommendations, particularly those concerning new drugs.

The authors of this volume have taken care that the information contained herein is accurate and compatible with the standards generally accepted at the time of publication. Nevertheless, it is difficult to ensure that all the information given is entirely accurate for all circumstances. The publisher and authors do not guarantee the contents of this book and disclaim any liability, loss, or damage incurred as a consequence, directly or indirectly, of the use and application of any of the contents of this volume.

The publisher's policy is to use permanent paper from mills that operate a sustainable forestry policy, and which has been manufactured from pulp processed using acid-free and elementary chlorine-free practices. Furthermore, the publisher ensures that the text paper and cover board used have met acceptable environmental accreditation standards.

CONTENTS

CONTRIBUTORS	ix
ACKNOWLEDGMENTS	x
HOW TO USE THIS BOOK	xii
ABBREVIATIONS	xiii
Case 1	1
Case 2	2
Case 3	3
Case 4	4
Case 5	5
Case 6	6
Case 7	7
Case 8	8
Case 9	9
Case 10	10
Case 11	11
Case 12	12
Case 13	13
Case 14	14
Case 15	15
Case 16	16
Case 17	17
Case 18	18
Case 19	19
Case 20	20
Case 21	21
Case 22	22
Case 23	23
Case 24	24
Case 25	25
Case 26	26
Case 27	27
Case 28	28
Case 29	29
Case 30	30

Case 31	31
Case 32	32
Case 33	33
Case 34	34
Case 35	35
Case 36	36
Case 37	37
Case 38	38
Case 39	39
Case 40	40
Case 41	41
Case 42	42
Case 43	43
Case 44	44
Case 45	45
Case 46	46
Case 47	47
Case 48	48
Case 49	49
Case 50	50
Case 51	51
Case 52	52
Case 53	53
Case 54	54
Case 55	55
Case 56	56
Case 57	57
Case 58	58
Case 59	59
Case 60	60
Case 61	61
Case 62	62
Case 63	63
Case 64	64
Case 65	65
Case 66	66

Case 67	67
Case 68	68
Case 69	69
Case 70	70
Case 71	71
Case 72	72
Case 73	73
Case 74	74
Case 75	75
Case 76	76
Case 77	77
Case 78	78
Case 79	79
Case 80	80
Case 81	81
Case 82	82
Case 83	83
Case 84	84
Case 85	85
Case 86	86
Case 87	87
Case 88	88
Case 89	89
Case 90	90
Case 91	91
Case 92	92
Case 93	93
Case 94	94
Case 95	95
Case 96	96
Case 97	97
Case 98	98
Case 99	99
Case 100	100
Case 101	101
Case 102	102

Case 103	103
Case 104	104
Case 105	105
Case 106	106
Case 107	107
Case 108	108
Case 109	109
Case 110	110
Case 111	111
Case 112	112
Case 113	113
Case 114	114
Case 115	115
Case 116	116

ANSWER KEY	117
Q&AS	119

CONTRIBUTORS

Ali Asghar Gamini, MD
Shiraz University School of Medicine, Class of 1994
Assistant Professor of Microbiology and Immunology, St. Luke's University School of Medicine

Alireza Khazaeizadeh, MD
Shiraz University School of Medicine, Class of 1995
Associate Professor, Department of Biochemistry, St. Luke's University School of Medicine

Chad Silverberg
Philadelphia College of Osteopathic Medicine, Class of 2004
Resident in Internal Medicine, Cleveland Clinic Foundation
Radiology Resident / Christiana Hospital (From 2005)

Hoang Nguyen, MD, MBA
Northwestern University, Class of 2001

Shalin Patel, MD
McGraw Medical Center, Northwestern University, Resident in Internal Medicine

Sonal Shah, MD
Ross University, Class of 2000

Vipal Soni, MD
UCLA School of Medicine, Class of 1999

Faculty Reviewer

Warren Levinson, MD, PHD
Professor of Microbiology and Immunology, UCSF School of Medicine

ACKNOWLEDGMENTS

Throughout the production of this book, we have had the support of many friends and colleagues. Special thanks to our support team including Andrea Fellows, Anastasia Anderson, Srishti Gupta, Anu Gupta, Mona Pall, Jonathan Kirsch and Chirag Amin. For prior contributions we thank Gianni Le Nguyen, Tarun Mathur, Alex Grimm, Sonia Santos and Elizabeth Sanders.

For submitting comments, corrections, editing, proofreading, and assistance across all of the vignette titles in all editions, we collectively thank:

Tara Adamovich, Carolyn Alexander, Kris Alden, Henry E. Aryan, Lynman Bacolor, Natalie Barteneva, Dean Bartholomew, Debashish Behera, Sumit Bhatia, Sanjay Bindra, Dave Brinton, Julianne Brown, Alexander Brownie, Tamara Callahan, David Canes, Bryan Casey, Aaron Caughey, Hebert Chen, Jonathan Cheng, Arnold Cheung, Arnold Chin, Simion Chiosea, Yoon Cho, Samuel Chung, Gretchen Conant, Vladimir Coric, Christopher Cosgrove, Ronald Cowan, Karekin R. Cunningham, A. Sean Dalley, Rama Dandamudi, Sunit Das, Ryan Armando Dave, John David, Emmanuel de la Cruz, Robert DeMello, Navneet Dhillon, Sharmila Dissanaike, David Donson, Adolf Etchegaray, Alea Eusebio, Priscilla A. Frase, David Frenz, Kristin Gaumer, Yohannes Gebreegziabher, Anil Gehi, Tony George, L.M. Gotanco, Parul Goyal, Alex Grimm, Rajeev Gupta, Ahmad Halim, Sue Hall, David Hasselbacher, Tamra Heimert, Michelle Higley, Dan Hoit, Eric Jackson, Tim Jackson, Sundar Jayaraman, Pei-Ni Jone, Aarchan Joshi, Rajni K. Jutla, Faiyaz Kapadi, Seth Karp, Aaron S. Kesselheim, Sana Khan, Andrew Pin-wei Ko, Francis Kong, Paul Konitzky, Warren S. Krackov, Benjamin H.S. Lau, Ann LaCasce, Connie Lee, Scott Lee, Guillermo Lehmann, Kevin Leung, Paul Levett, Warren Levinson, Eric Ley, Ken Lin, Pavel Lobanov, J. Mark Maddox, Aram Mardian, Samir Mehta, Gil Melmed, Joe Messina, Robert Mosca, Sandra Mun, Michael Murphy, Vivek Nandkarni, Siva Naraynan, Carvell Nguyen, Linh Nguyen, Deanna Nobleza, Craig Nodurft, George Noumi, Darin T. Okuda, Adam L. Palance, Paul Pamphrus, Jinha Park, Sonny Patel, Ricardo Pietrobon, Riva L. Rahl, Aashita Randeria, Rachan Reddy, Beatriu Reig, Marilou Reyes, Jeremy Richmon, Tai Roe, Rick Roller, Rajiv Roy, Diego Ruiz, Anthony Russell, Sanjay Sahgal, Urmimala Sarkar, John Schilling, Isabell Schmitt, Daren Schuhmacher, Sonal Shah, Edie Shen, Justin Smith, John Stulak, Lillian Su, Julie Sundaram, Rita Suri, Seth Sweetser, Antonio Talayero, Merita Tan, Mark Tanaka, Eric Taylor, Jess Thompson, Indi Trehan, Raymond Turner, Okafo Uchenna, Eric Uyguanco, Richa Varma, John Wages, Alan Wang, Eunice Wang, Andy Weiss, Amy Williams, Brian Yang, Hany Zaky, Ashraf Zaman and David Zipf.

Please let us know if your name has been missed or misspelled and we will be happy to make the update in the next edition.

For generously contributing images to the entire Underground Clinical Vignette Step 1 series, we collectively thank the staff at Blackwell Publishing in Oxford, Boston, and Berlin as well as:

- Axford, J. Medicine. Osney Mead: Blackwell Science Ltd, 1996. Figures 2.14, 2.15, 2.16, 2.27, 2.28, 2.31, 2.35, 2.36, 2.38, 2.43, 2.65a, 2.65b, 2.65c, 2.103b, 2.105b, 3.20b, 3.21, 8.27, 8.27b, 8.77b, 8.77c, 10.81b, 10.96a, 12.28a, 14.6, 14.16, 14.50.

- Bannister B, Begg N, Gillespie S. Infectious Disease, 2nd Edition. Osney Mead: Blackwell Science Ltd, 2000. Figures 2.8, 3.4, 5.28, 18.10, W5.32, W5.6.

- Berg D. Advanced Clinical Skills and Physical Diagnosis. Blackwell Science Ltd., 1999. Figures 7.10, 7.12, 7.13, 7.2, 7.3, 7.7, 7.8, 7.9, 8.1, 8.2, 8.4, 8.5, 9.2, 10.2, 11.3, 11.5, 12.6.

- Cuschieri A, Hennessy TPJ, Greenhalgh RM, Rowley DA, Grace PA. Clinical Surgery. Osney Mead: Blackwell Science Ltd, 1996. Figures 13.19, 18.22, 18.33.

- Gillespie SH, Bamford K. *Medical Microbiology and Infection at a Glance.* Osney Mead.: Blackwell Science Ltd, 2000, Figures 20, 23.

- Ginsberg L. Lecture Notes on Neurology, 7th Edition. Osney Mead: Blackwell Science Ltd, 1999. Figures 12.3, 18.3, 18.3b.

- Elliott T, Hastings M, Desselberger U. Lecture Notes on Medical Microbiology, 3rd Edition. Osney Mead: Blackwell Science Ltd, 1997. Figures 2, 5, 7, 8, 9, 11, 12, 14, 15, 16, 17, 19, 20, 25, 26, 27, 29, 30, 34, 35, 52.

- Mehta AB, Hoffbrand AV. Haematology at a Glance. Osney Mead: Blackwell Science Ltd, 2000. Figures 22.1, 22.2, 22.3.

HOW TO USE THIS BOOK

This series was originally developed to address the increasing number of clinical vignette questions on medical examinations, including the USMLE Step 1 and Step 2.

Each UCV 1 book uses a series of approximately 100 "supra-prototypical" cases as a way to condense testable facts and associations. The clinical vignettes in this series are designed to give added emphasis to pathogenesis, epidemiology, management and complications. Although each case tends to present all the signs, symptoms, and diagnostic findings for a particular illness, patients generally will not present with such a "complete" picture either clinically or on a medical examination. Cases are not meant to simulate a potential real patient or an exam vignette. All the boldfaced "buzzwords" are for learning purposes and are not necessarily expected to be found in any one patient with the disease.

Definitions of selected important terms are placed within the vignettes in (small caps) in parentheses. Other parenthetical remarks often refer to the pathophysiology or mechanism of disease. The format should also help students learn to present cases succinctly during oral "bullet" presentations on clinical rotations. The cases are meant to serve as a condensed review, not as a primary reference. The information provided in this book has been prepared with a great deal of thought and careful research. This book should not, however, be considered as your sole source of information. Corrections, suggestions and submissions of new cases are encouraged and will be acknowledged and incorporated when appropriate in future editions.

We hope that you find the *Blackwell Underground Clinical Vignettes* series informative and useful. We welcome feedback and suggestions you have about this book, or any published by Blackwell Publishing.

Please e-mail us at medfeedback@bos.blackwellpublishing.com.

ABBREVIATIONS

ABGs	arterial blood gases
ABPA	allergic bronchopulmonary aspergillosis
ACA	anticardiolipin antibody
ACE	angiotensin-converting enzyme
ACL	anterior cruciate ligament
ACTH	adrenocorticotropic hormone
AD	adjustment disorder
ADA	adenosine deaminase
ADD	attention deficit disorder
ADH	antidiuretic hormone
ADHD	attention deficit hyperactivity disorder
ADP	adenosine diphosphate
AFO	ankle-foot orthosis
AFP	α-fetoprotein
AIDS	acquired immunodeficiency syndrome
ALL	acute lymphocytic leukemia
ALS	amyotrophic lateral sclerosis
ALT	alanine aminotransferase
AML	acute myelogenous leukemia
ANA	antinuclear antibody
Angio	angiography
AP	anteroposterior
APKD	adult polycystic kidney disease
aPTT	activated partial thromboplastin time
ARDS	adult respiratory distress syndrome
5-ASA	5-aminosalicylic acid
ASCA	antibodies to *Saccharomyces cerevisiae*
ASO	antistreptolysin O
AST	aspartate aminotransferase
ATLL	adult T-cell leukemia/lymphoma
ATPase	adenosine triphosphatase
AV	arteriovenous, atrioventricular
AZT	azidothymidine (zidovudine)
BAL	British antilewisite (dimercaprol)
BCG	bacille Calmette-Guérin
BE	barium enema
BP	blood pressure
BPH	benign prostatic hypertrophy
BUN	blood urea nitrogen
CABG	coronary artery bypass grafting
CAD	coronary artery disease
CaEDTA	calcium edetate
CALLA	common acute lymphoblastic leukemia antigen
cAMP	cyclic adenosine monophosphate
C-ANCA	cytoplasmic antineutrophil cytoplasmic antibody
CBC	complete blood count

CBD	common bile duct
CCU	cardiac care unit
CD	cluster of differentiation
2-CdA	2-chlorodeoxyadenosine
CEA	carcinoembryonic antigen
CFTR	cystic fibrosis transmembrane conductance regulator
cGMP	cyclic guanosine monophosphate
CHF	congestive heart failure
CK	creatine kinase
CK-MB	creatine kinase, MB fraction
CLL	chronic lymphocytic leukemia
CML	chronic myelogenous leukemia
CMV	cytomegalovirus
CN	cranial nerve
CNS	central nervous system
COPD	chronic obstructive pulmonary disease
COX	cyclooxygenase
CP	cerebellopontine
CPAP	continuous positive airway pressure
CPK	creatine phosphokinase
CPPD	calcium pyrophosphate dihydrate
CPR	cardiopulmonary resuscitation
CREST	calcinosis, Raynaud's phenomenon, esophageal involvement, sclerodactyly, telangiectasia (syndrome)
CRP	C-reactive protein
CSF	cerebrospinal fluid
CSOM	chronic suppurative otitis media
CT	cardiac transplant, computed tomography
CVA	cerebrovascular accident
CXR	chest x-ray
d4T	didehydrodeoxythymidine (stavudine)
DCS	decompression sickness
DDH	developmental dysplasia of the hip
ddI	dideoxyinosine (didanosine)
DES	diethylstilbestrol
DEXA	dual-energy x-ray absorptiometry
DHEAS	dehydroepiandrosterone sulfate
DIC	disseminated intravascular coagulation
DIF	direct immunofluorescence
DIP	distal interphalangeal (joint)
DKA	diabetic ketoacidosis
DL_{CO}	diffusing capacity of carbon monoxide
DMSA	2,3-dimercaptosuccinic acid
DNA	deoxyribonucleic acid
DNase	deoxyribonuclease
2,3-DPG	2,3-diphosphoglycerate

dsDNA	double-stranded DNA
DSM	Diagnostic and Statistical Manual
dsRNA	double-stranded RNA
DTP	diphtheria, tetanus, pertussis (vaccine)
DTPA	diethylenetriamine-penta-acetic acid
DTs	delirium tremens
DVT	deep venous thrombosis
EBV	Epstein-Barr virus
ECG	electrocardiography
Echo	echocardiography
ECM	erythema chronicum migrans
ECT	electroconvulsive therapy
EEG	electroencephalography
EF	ejection fraction, elongation factor
EGD	esophagogastroduodenoscopy
EHEC	enterohemorrhagic *E. coli*
EIA	enzyme immunoassay
ELISA	enzyme-linked immunosorbent assay
EM	electron microscopy
EMG	electromyography
ENT	ears, nose, and throat
EPVE	early prosthetic valve endocarditis
ER	emergency room
ERCP	endoscopic retrograde cholangiopancreatography
ERT	estrogen replacement therapy
ESR	erythrocyte sedimentation rate
ETEC	enterotoxigenic *E. coli*
EtOH	ethanol
FAP	familial adenomatous polyposis
FEV_1	forced expiratory volume in 1 second
FH	familial hypercholesterolemia
FNA	fine-needle aspiration
FSH	follicle-stimulating hormone
FTA-ABS	fluorescent treponemal antibody absorption test
FVC	forced vital capacity
G6PD	glucose-6-phosphate dehydrogenase
GABA	gamma-aminobutyric acid
GERD	gastroesophageal reflux disease
GFR	glomerular filtration rate
GGT	gamma-glutamyltransferase
GH	growth hormone
GI	gastrointestinal
GnRH	gonadotropin-releasing hormone
GU	genitourinary
GVHD	graft-versus-host disease
HAART	highly active antiretroviral therapy

HAV	hepatitis A virus
Hb	hemoglobin
HbA-1C	hemoglobin A-1C
HBsAg	hepatitis B surface antigen
HBV	hepatitis B virus
hCG	human chorionic gonadotropin
HCO_3	bicarbonate
Hct	hematocrit
HCV	hepatitis C virus
HDL	high-density lipoprotein
HDL-C	high-density lipoprotein-cholesterol
HEENT	head, eyes, ears, nose, and throat (exam)
HELLP	hemolysis, elevated LFTs, low platelets (syndrome)
HFMD	hand, foot, and mouth disease
HGPRT	hypoxanthine-guanine phosphoribosyltransferase
5-HIAA	5-hydroxyindoleacetic acid
HIDA	hepato-iminodiacetic acid (scan)
HIV	human immunodeficiency virus
HLA	human leukocyte antigen
HMG-CoA	hydroxymethylglutaryl-coenzyme A
HMP	hexose monophosphate
HPI	history of present illness
HPV	human papillomavirus
HR	heart rate
HRIG	human rabies immune globulin
HRS	hepatorenal syndrome
HRT	hormone replacement therapy
HSG	hysterosalpingography
HSV	herpes simplex virus
HTLV	human T-cell leukemia virus
HUS	hemolytic-uremic syndrome
HVA	homovanillic acid
ICP	intracranial pressure
ICU	intensive care unit
ID/CC	identification and chief complaint
IDDM	insulin-dependent diabetes mellitus
IFA	immunofluorescent antibody
Ig	immunoglobulin
IGF	insulin-like growth factor
IHSS	idiopathic hypertrophic subaortic stenosis
IM	intramuscular
IMA	inferior mesenteric artery
INH	isoniazid
INR	International Normalized Ratio
IP_3	inositol 1,4,5-triphosphate
IPF	idiopathic pulmonary fibrosis

ITP	idiopathic thrombocytopenic purpura
IUD	intrauterine device
IV	intravenous
IVC	inferior vena cava
IVIG	intravenous immunoglobulin
IVP	intravenous pyelography
JRA	juvenile rheumatoid arthritis
JVP	jugular venous pressure
KOH	potassium hydroxide
KUB	kidney, ureter, bladder
LCM	lymphocytic choriomeningitis
LDH	lactate dehydrogenase
LDL	low-density lipoprotein
LE	lupus erythematosus (cell)
LES	lower esophageal sphincter
LFTs	liver function tests
LH	luteinizing hormone
LMN	lower motor neuron
LP	lumbar puncture
LPVE	late prosthetic valve endocarditis
L/S	lecithin-sphingomyelin (ratio)
LSD	lysergic acid diethylamide
LT	labile toxin
LV	left ventricular
LVH	left ventricular hypertrophy
Lytes	electrolytes
Mammo	mammography
MAO	monoamine oxidase (inhibitor)
MCP	metacarpophalangeal (joint)
MCTD	mixed connective tissue disorder
MCV	mean corpuscular volume
MEN	multiple endocrine neoplasia
MI	myocardial infarction
MIBG	meta-iodobenzylguanidine (radioisotope)
MMR	measles, mumps, rubella (vaccine)
MPGN	membranoproliferative glomerulonephritis
MPS	mucopolysaccharide
MPTP	1-methyl-4-phenyl-tetrahydropyridine
MR	magnetic resonance (imaging)
mRNA	messenger ribonucleic acid
MRSA	methicillin-resistant S. aureus
MTP	metatarsophalangeal (joint)
NAD	nicotinamide adenine dinucleotide
NADP	nicotinamide adenine dinucleotide phosphate
NADPH	reduced nicotinamide adenine dinucleotide phosphate
NF	neurofibromatosis

NIDDM	non-insulin-dependent diabetes mellitus
NNRTI	non-nucleoside reverse transcriptase inhibitor
NO	nitric oxide
NPO	nil per os (nothing by mouth)
NSAID	nonsteroidal anti-inflammatory drug
Nuc	nuclear medicine
NYHA	New York Heart Association
OB	obstetric
OCD	obsessive-compulsive disorder
OCPs	oral contraceptive pills
OR	operating room
PA	posteroanterior
PABA	para-aminobenzoic acid
PAN	polyarteritis nodosa
P-ANCA	perinuclear antineutrophil cytoplasmic antibody
Pa_{O_2}	partial pressure of oxygen in arterial blood
PAS	periodic acid Schiff
PAT	paroxysmal atrial tachycardia
PBS	peripheral blood smear
P_{CO_2}	partial pressure of carbon dioxide
PCOM	posterior communicating (artery)
PCOS	polycystic ovarian syndrome
PCP	phencyclidine
PCR	polymerase chain reaction
PCT	porphyria cutanea tarda
PCTA	percutaneous coronary transluminal angioplasty
PCV	polycythemia vera
PDA	patent ductus arteriosus
PDGF	platelet-derived growth factor
PE	physical exam
PEFR	peak expiratory flow rate
PEG	polyethylene glycol
PEPCK	phosphoenolpyruvate carboxykinase
PET	positron emission tomography
PFTs	pulmonary function tests
PID	pelvic inflammatory disease
PIP	proximal interphalangeal (joint)
PKU	phenylketonuria
PMDD	premenstrual dysphoric disorder
PML	progressive multifocal leukoencephalopathy
PMN	polymorphonuclear (leukocyte)
PNET	primitive neuroectodermal tumor
PNH	paroxysmal nocturnal hemoglobinuria
P_{O_2}	partial pressure of oxygen
PPD	purified protein derivative (of tuberculosis)
PPH	primary postpartum hemorrhage

PRA	panel reactive antibody
PROM	premature rupture of membranes
PSA	prostate-specific antigen
PSS	progressive systemic sclerosis
PT	prothrombin time
PTH	parathyroid hormone
PTSD	post-traumatic stress disorder
PTT	partial thromboplastin time
PUVA	psoralen ultraviolet A
PVC	premature ventricular contraction
RA	rheumatoid arthritis
RAIU	radioactive iodine uptake
RAST	radioallergosorbent test
RBC	red blood cell
REM	rapid eye movement
RES	reticuloendothelial system
RFFIT	rapid fluorescent focus inhibition test
RFTs	renal function tests
RHD	rheumatic heart disease
RNA	ribonucleic acid
RNP	ribonucleoprotein
RPR	rapid plasma reagin
RR	respiratory rate
RSV	respiratory syncytial virus
RUQ	right upper quadrant
RV	residual volume
Sao_2	oxygen saturation in arterial blood
SBFT	small bowel follow-through
SCC	squamous cell carcinoma
SCID	severe combined immunodeficiency
SERM	selective estrogen receptor modulator
SGOT	serum glutamic-oxaloacetic transaminase
SIADH	syndrome of inappropriate antidiuretic hormone
SIDS	sudden infant death syndrome
SLE	systemic lupus erythematosus
SMA	superior mesenteric artery
SSPE	subacute sclerosing panencephalitis
SSRI	selective serotonin reuptake inhibitor
ST	stable toxin
STD	sexually transmitted disease
T2W	T2-weighted (MRI)
T_3	triiodothyronine
T_4	thyroxine
TAH-BSO	total abdominal hysterectomy–bilateral salpingo-oophorectomy
TB	tuberculosis
TCA	tricyclic antidepressant

TCC	transitional cell carcinoma
TDT	terminal deoxytransferase
TFTs	thyroid function tests
TGF	transforming growth factor
THC	tetrahydrocannabinol
TIA	transient ischemic attack
TLC	total lung capacity
TMP-SMX	trimethoprim-sulfamethoxazole
tPA	tissue plasminogen activator
TP-HA	*Treponema pallidum* hemagglutination assay
TPP	thiamine pyrophosphate
TRAP	tartrate-resistant acid phosphatase
tRNA	transfer ribonucleic acid
TSH	thyroid-stimulating hormone
TSS	toxic shock syndrome
TTP	thrombotic thrombocytopenic purpura
TURP	transurethral resection of the prostate
TXA	thromboxane A
UA	urinalysis
UDCA	ursodeoxycholic acid
UGI	upper GI
UPPP	uvulopalatopharyngoplasty
URI	upper respiratory infection
US	ultrasound
UTI	urinary tract infection
UV	ultraviolet
VDRL	Venereal Disease Research Laboratory
VIN	vulvar intraepithelial neoplasia
VIP	vasoactive intestinal polypeptide
VLDL	very low density lipoprotein
VMA	vanillylmandelic acid
V/Q	ventilation/perfusion (ratio)
VRE	vancomycin-resistant enterococcus
VS	vital signs
VSD	ventricular septal defect
vWF	von Willebrand's factor
VZV	varicella-zoster virus
WAGR	Wilms' tumor, aniridia, genitourinary abnormalities, mental retardation (syndrome)
WBC	white blood cell
WHI	Women's Health Initiative
WPW	Wolff-Parkinson-White syndrome
XR	x-ray
ZN	Ziehl-Neelsen (stain)

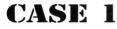

ID/CC A 34-year-old male presents to his primary care physician with a hard, red, painless **swelling** on his left **mandible** that has slowly been growing over the past few weeks and has now begun to **drain pus.**

HPI The patient **recently had a tooth extraction.**

PE No acute distress; no other significant findings.

Labs Gram stain of exudate reveals **branching gram-positive filaments** and characteristic **"sulfur granules"**; non-acid-fast and anaerobic (distinguishes actinomyces from *Nocardia*).

Imaging XR: no bony destruction.

Gross Pathology **Sinus tracts** from region of infection to surface with granular exudate.

Micro Pathology Granulation tissue and fibrosis surrounding a central suppurative necrosis; granulation tissue may also enclose foamy histiocytes and plasma cells.

Treatment Ampicillin followed by amoxicillin or penicillin G followed by oral penicillin V and, if necessary, surgical drainage and removal of necrotic tissue.

Discussion *Actinomyces israelii* is a part of the normal flora of the mouth (crypts of tonsils and tartar of teeth), so most patients have a history of surgery or trauma. There is **no person-to-person spread.** Actinomycosis is a chronic suppurative infection and can also involve the abdomen or lungs, especially following a penetrating trauma such as a bullet wound or an intestinal perforation. Pelvic disease is associated with IUD use. Spread occurs contiguously, not hematogenously.

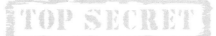

CASE 2

ID/CC A 25-year-old **IV drug abuser** presents with a **high fever** with chills, malaise, a productive cough, hemoptysis, and right-sided pleuritic chest pain.

HPI He also reports multiple skin infections at injection sites.

PE VS: fever. PE: **stigmata of intravenous drug abuse** at multiple injection sites; skin infections; thrombosed peripheral veins; **splenomegaly and pulsatile hepatomegaly**; **ejection systolic murmur**, increasing with inspiration, heard in tricuspid area.

Labs CBC: normochromic, normocytic anemia. UA: microscopic hematuria. Blood culture yields *Staphylococcus aureus*.

Imaging Echo: presence of **vegetations on tricuspid valve** and **tricuspid incompetence**. CXR: consolidation.

Treatment **High-dose intravenous penicillinase-resistant penicillin** in combination with an **aminoglycoside**. If the isolated *S. aureus* strain is **methicillin resistant, vancomycin** is the drug of choice.

Discussion In drug addicts, the **tricuspid valve** is the site of infection more frequently (55%) than the aortic valve (35%) or the mitral valve (30%); these findings contrast markedly with the rarity of right-sided involvement in cases of infective endocarditis that are not associated with drug abuse. *Staphylococcus aureus* is responsible for the majority of cases. Certain organisms have a predilection for particular valves in cases of addict-associated endocarditis; for example, enterococci, other streptococcal species, and non-albicans *Candida* organisms predominantly affect the valves of the left side of the heart, while *S. aureus* infects valves on both the right and the left side of the heart. *Pseudomonas* organisms are associated with biventricular and multiple-valve infection in addicts. Complications of endocarditis include congestive heart failure, ruptured valve cusp, myocardial infarction, and myocardial abscess.

ID/CC A **7-month-old** girl is brought to the pediatric clinic with **wheezing**, respiratory difficulty, and nasal congestion of 3 hours' duration.

HPI She has had rhinorrhea, fever, and cough and had been sneezing for 2 days prior to her visit to the clinic.

PE VS: **tachypnea**. PE: **nasal flaring**; mild central **cyanosis**; accessory muscle use during respiration; hyperexpansion of chest; expiratory and inspiratory wheezes; **rhonchi** over both lung fields.

Labs CBC/PBS: relative **lymphocytosis**. ABGs: **hypoxemia with mild hypercapnia**. **Respiratory syncytial virus (RSV)** demonstrated on viral culture of throat swab.

Imaging CXR: **hyperinflation**; segmental **atelectasis**; **interstitial infiltrates**.

Micro Pathology Severe bronchiolitis produces bronchiolar epithelial necrosis, lymphocytic infiltrate, and alveolar exudates.

Treatment Humidified oxygen, bronchodilators, aerosolized **ribavirin**.

Discussion **RSV is the most common cause of bronchiolitis in infants** under 2 years of age; other viral causes include parainfluenza, influenza, and adenovirus. RSV shedding may last 2 or more weeks in children.

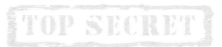

ID/CC A 25-year-old woman visits her family physician because of marked **burning pain while urinating** (DYSURIA), **increased frequency of urination** with **small amounts of urine** (POLLAKIURIA), and passage of a few drops of **blood-stained** debris at the end of urination (HEMATURIA).

HPI She got married 2 weeks ago and has **just returned from her honeymoon.**

PE VS: no fever; BP normal. PE: no edema; no costovertebral angle tenderness; moderate suprapubic tenderness with **urgency.**

Labs UA: urine collected in two glasses; second glass more turbid and blood-stained; urine sediment reveals RBCs and WBCs; **no RBC or WBC casts**; Gram stain of urine sediment reveals **gram-negative bacilli**; *Escherichia coli* in significant colony count (> 100,000) on urine culture.

Treatment Oral antibiotics (Bactrim, fluoroquinolone); adequate hydration.

Discussion *E. coli* is the most common pathogen; *Proteus, Klebsiella, Staphylococcus saprophyticus*, and *Enterococcus* are other common bacteria causing cystitis. Hemorrhagic cystitis may result from adenoviral infection.

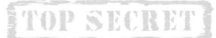

CASE 5

BACTERIOLOGY

ID/CC
An **8-year-old** female presents with pain and swelling of her knee joints, elbows, and lower limbs along with **fever** for the past 2 weeks; she also complains of shortness of breath (DYSPNEA) on exertion.

HPI
The patient had a **sore throat 2 weeks ago.**

PE
VS: fever. PE: **blanching, ring-shaped erythematous rash over trunk and proximal extremities** (ERYTHEMA MARGINATUM); **subcutaneous nodules** at occiput and below extensor tendons in elbow; **swelling with redness of both knee joints and elbows** (POLYARTHRITIS); painfully restricted movement; pedal edema; increased JVP; high-frequency apical systolic murmur with radiation to axillae (**mitral valve insufficiency due to carditis**); bilateral fine inspiratory basal crepitant rales; mild, tender hepatomegaly.

Labs
CBC: leukocytosis. *Streptococcus pyogenes* on throat swab; markedly **elevated ASO titers; elevated ESR; elevated C-reactive protein (CRP);** negative blood culture. ECG: **prolonged P-R interval.**

Imaging
CXR: cardiomegaly; increased pulmonary vascular markings. Echo: vegetations over mitral valve with regurgitation.

Gross Pathology
Acute form characterized by **endo-, myo-, and pericarditis** (PANCARDITIS); chronic form characterized by fibrous scarring with calcification and mitral stenosis with verrucous fibrin deposits.

Micro Pathology
Myocardial muscle fiber necrosis enmeshed in collagen; characteristic finding is fibrinoid necrosis surrounded by **perivascular accumulation of mononuclear inflammatory cells** (ASCHOFF CELLS).

Treatment
Penicillin to eradicate streptococcal infection; high-dose salicylates for analgesic and anti-inflammatory effect; rest and corticosteroids if there is evidence of carditis resulting in congestive failure; long-term penicillin prophylaxis.

Discussion
Acute rheumatic fever is a sequela of upper respiratory infection with group A, β-hemolytic streptococcus; it causes **autoimmune** damage to several organs, primarily the heart. The systemic effects of acute rheumatic fever are immune mediated and are secondary to cross-reactivity of host antistreptococcal antibodies.

5

ID/CC   A 35-year-old woman complains of fever and **pain in the face** and **upper teeth** (maxillary sinus), especially while leaning forward.

HPI   She has had a chronic cough, **nasal congestion, and discharge** for the past few months.

PE   VS: fever. PE: halitosis; greenish-yellow **postnasal discharge**; bilateral **boggy nasal mucosa**; bilateral percussion tenderness and **erythema over zygomatic arch; clouding of sinuses by transillumination**; dental and cranial nerve exams normal.

Labs   Nasal cultures reveal *Streptococcus pneumoniae*.

Imaging   CT, sinus: partial opacification of maxillary sinus with air-fluid level.

Gross Pathology   Erythematous and edematous nasal mucosa.

Micro Pathology   Presence of organisms and leukocytes in mucosa.

Treatment   Oral decongestants; amoxicillin, Bactrim, or fluoroquinolone.

Discussion   Other pathogens include other streptococci, *Haemophilus influenzae*, and *Moraxella*. The obstruction of ostia in the anterior ethmoid and middle meatal complex by retained secretions, mucosal edema, or polyps promotes sinusitis. *Staphylococcus aureus* and gram-negative species may cause chronic sinusitis. Fungal sinusitis may mimic chronic bacterial sinusitis. Complications include orbital cellulitis and abscesses.

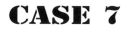

ID/CC
A 30-year-old male goes to the emergency room because of **dyspnea,** cyanosis, hemoptysis, and chest pain.

HPI
He has had a high fever, malaise, and a **nonproductive cough** for 1 week. The patient is a **sheep farmer** who remembers having been treated for **dark black skin lesions** in the past.

PE
VS: fever. PE: dyspnea; cyanosis; bilateral rales heard over lungs.

Labs
CBC: normal. Negative blood and sputum cultures; diagnosis of anthrax confirmed by fourfold increase in indirect microhemagglutination titer.

Imaging
CXR: mediastinal widening. CT, chest: evidence of "**hemorrhagic mediastinitis.**"

Gross Pathology
Patchy consolidation; vesicular papules covered by **black eschar.**

Micro Pathology
Lungs show fibrinous exudate with many organisms but few PMNs.

Treatment
Isolate and treat with IV penicillin G, doxycycline, or fluoroquinolones; antibiotics for postexposure prophylaxis of contacts.

Discussion
Anthrax is caused by infection with *Bacillus anthracis*. A cell-free anthrax vaccine is available to protect those employed in industries associated with a high risk of anthrax transmission (farmers, veterinarians, tannery or wool workers).

CASE 8

ID/CC A 50-year-old **alcoholic male** presents with a high-grade **fever, cough, copious, foul-smelling sputum**, and pleuritic right-sided chest pain.

HPI His wife reports that he was brought home in a **semiconscious state a few days ago**, when he was found lying on the roadside heavily under the influence of alcohol.

PE VS: fever. PE: signs of consolidation elicited over **right middle and lower pulmonary lobes**.

Labs Sputum reveals abundant PMN leukocytes and mixed oral flora; **culture yields *Bacteroides melaninogenicus (Prevotella melaninogenica)* and other *Bacteroides* species, *Fusobacterium*, microaerophilic streptococci**, and *Peptostreptococcus*.

Imaging CXR: consolidation involving apical segment of right lower lobe and posterior segments of middle lobe; large cavity with air-fluid level (ABSCESS) also seen.

Treatment Clindamycin.

Discussion Alcoholism, drug abuse, administration of sedatives or anesthesia, head trauma, and seizures or other neurologic disorders are most often responsible for the development of aspiration pneumonia. Because anaerobes are the dominant flora of the upper GI tract (outnumbering aerobic or facultative bacteria by 10 to 1), they are the dominant organisms in aspiration pneumonia; of particular importance are *Bacteroides melaninogenicus (Prevotella melaninogenica)* and other *Bacteroides* species (slender, pleomorphic, pale gram-negative rods), *Fusobacterium nucleatum* (slender gram-negative rods with pointed ends), and anaerobic or microaerophilic streptococci and *Peptostreptococcus* (small gram-positive cocci in chains or clumps).

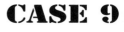
ID/CC   A 38-year-old **HIV-positive** male is admitted to the hospital with **fever, rigors, night sweats, and diarrhea.**

HPI   He reports excessive weight loss over the past few weeks. He was treated for *Pneumocystis* **pneumonia** a few weeks ago and still reports a persistent productive cough.

PE   VS: fever. PE: patient is extremely emaciated; hepatosplenomegaly and lymphadenopathy noted.

Labs   CD4+ count < 50/cc; *Mycobacterium avium-intracellulare* isolated on blood culture; smears of tissues obtained from lymph nodes, bone marrow, spleen, liver, and lungs reveal evidence of acid-fast bacilli, and cultures yield *M. avium*; intestinal infection with *M. avium* proven by culture of stools and colonic biopsy specimens.

Imaging   CT, abdomen: hepatosplenomegaly; retroperitoneal lymphadenopathy; bowel mucosal fold thickening.

Micro Pathology   Despite the presence of many mycobacteria and macrophages, well-formed granulomas were typically absent due to **profound impairment of cell-mediated immunity.**

Treatment Multiagent antibiotic therapy combining one macrolide (e.g., clarithromycin) with ethambutol, rifampin, clofazimine, or quinolones.

Discussion *Mycobacterium avium* complex is now the **most frequent opportunistic bacterial infection in patients with AIDS**; it typically occurs late in the course of the syndrome, when other opportunistic infections and neoplasia have already occurred. Prophylaxis against *M. avium-intracellulare* is recommended in AIDS patients with a CD4+ count of < 100/mm^3 (administer azithromycin, clarithromycin, or rifabutin).

ID/CC	A 20-year-old male from **India** presents to the ER with **severe nausea and vomiting**.
HPI	Careful history reveals that 2 hours ago he ate some **unrefrigerated fried rice** that his wife had cooked the night before. He does not complain of any fever or diarrhea (may or may not be present).
PE	VS: no fever. PE: mild dehydration; diffuse mild abdominal tenderness.
Labs	Fecal staining reveals no RBCs, WBCs, or parasites; *Bacillus cereus,* **a gram-positive rod**, isolated from vomitus and stool and shown to produce the **emetogenic enterotoxin**.
Treatment	Supportive.
Discussion	*Bacillus cereus* causes two distinct syndromes: a **diarrheal form** (mediated by an *Escherichia coli* LT-type enterotoxin with an incubation period of 8 to 16 hours; caused by meats and vegetables) and an **emetic form** (mediated by a *Staphylococcus aureus*-type enterotoxin with an incubation period of 1 to 8 hours; caused by fried rice). Proper food handling and refrigeration of boiled rice are largely preventive.

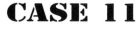

CASE 11

ID/CC
A 25-year-old **recently married woman** is concerned about a scanty, offensively **malodorous vaginal discharge**.

HPI
She states that the discharge is **thin, grayish-white, and foul-smelling**. She does not complain of vulvar pruritus or soreness.

PE
Pelvic exam confirms presence of a homogenous, grayish-white, watery discharge adherent to the vaginal walls that yields a **"fishy" odor when mixed with KOH**; no injection and excoriation of the vulva, vagina, or cervix.

Labs
Vaginal pH > 5; saline smear reveals presence of **characteristic "clue cells"** (squamous epithelial cells with smudged borders due to adherent bacteria).

Treatment
Single dose of **metronidazole** (2 g) effective in treating the infection. Oral clindamycin is an alternative drug.

Discussion
Although bacterial vaginitis was originally thought to be caused by *Gardnerella vaginalis*, this organism is now recognized to be part of the normal vaginal flora. Bacterial vaginosis is now known to result from a **synergistic interaction of bacteria** in which the normal *Lactobacillus* species in the vagina is ultimately replaced by **high concentrations of anaerobic bacteria**, including *Bacteroides, Peptostreptococcus, Peptococcus,* and *Mobiluncus* **species** along with a markedly greater number of *G. vaginalis* organisms than is encountered in normal vaginal secretions. Bacterial vaginosis is known to increase the risk of pelvic inflammatory disease, chorioamnionitis, and premature birth.

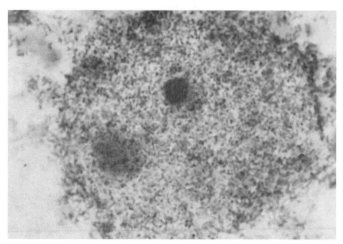

Figure 011 Epithelial cell covered with bacteria.

ID/CC   A 30-year-old male who recently emigrated from **Peru** presents with an extensive **nodular skin eruption**, mild arthralgias, and occasional fever.

HPI   One month ago, the patient had a high-grade **fever** that was accompanied by excessive weakness, dyspnea, and passage of **cola-colored urine**; the fever subsided after 2 weeks, but his weakness has progressed since that time.

PE   Pallor; mild icterus; extensive skin rash comprising **purplish nodular lesions** of varying sizes seen on face, trunk, and limbs; mild hepatosplenomegaly; funduscopy reveals **retinal hemorrhages**.

Labs   **Intraerythrocytic coccobacillary**-form bacteria visible in thick and thin films stained with Giemsa; **bacteria** seen and **isolated from skin lesions**; indirect serum bilirubin elevated. PBS: macrocytic, hypochromic anemia with polychromasia; marked reticulocytosis (due to hemolytic anemia); Coombs' test negative.

Micro Pathology   Skin biopsy of vascular skin lesions reveals endothelial proliferation and histiocytic hyperplasia; electron microscopy of verrucous tissue shows *Bartonella bacilliformis* in interstitial tissue.

Treatment   **Penicillin**, **erythromycin**, **norfloxacin**, and **tetracycline** are effective; rifampicin is indicated for treatment of verrucous forms.

Discussion   Bartonellosis is a sandfly-borne bacterial disease occurring only on the **western coast of South America** at high altitudes; the causative agent is a motile, pleomorphic bacillus, *Bartonella bacilliformis*. Two stages of the disease are recognized: an **initial febrile stage** associated with a **hemolytic anemia** (OROYA FEVER) and a later cutaneous stage characterized by **hemangiomatous nodules** (VERRUGA PERUANA).

ID/CC

A 25-year-old male presents with sudden-onset **double vision** (DIPLOPIA), **dry mouth, weakness, dysarthria**, and **dysphagia**.

HPI

He has no previous history of episodic weakness or of dog or tick bites (vs. myasthenia gravis, rabies, or Lyme disease). Last night, he ate some **home-canned food**.

PE

VS: no fever. PE: patient alert; ptosis; bilateral **third and tenth cranial nerve palsy**; symmetric **flaccid paralysis** of all four limbs; deep tendon reflexes reduced; no sensory loss seen; decreased bowel sounds.

Labs

Botulinum toxin detected in patient's serum and canned-food sample with specific antiserum.

Treatment

Antitoxin; close monitoring of respiratory status; intubation for respiratory failure.

Discussion

The disease is characterized by gradual return of muscle strength in most cases. Botulinum toxin is a zinc metalloprotease that cleaves specific components of synaptic vesicle docking and fusion complexes, thus **inhibiting the release of acetylcholine at the neuromuscular junction**. The disease in adults is due to **ingestion of the toxin** rather than to bacterial infection. Botulism is also seen in infants secondary to the ingestion of *Clostridium botulinum* spores in **honey**.

CASE 14

ID/CC A 10-year-old female presents with a **high fever, headache, vomiting,** and impaired consciousness.

HPI She suffered a generalized **seizure** about 45 minutes ago. She was previously diagnosed with **cyanotic congenital heart disease** (ventricular septal defect with Eisenmenger's syndrome).

PE VS: fever. PE: altered sensorium; **papilledema**; nuchal rigidity; clubbing; **central cyanosis**; cardiac auscultation suggestive of VSD with severe pulmonary arterial hypertension.

Labs Blood culture reveals **mixed infection** with *Bacteroides*, microaerophilic streptococci, *Staphylococcus aureus*, and *Klebsiella*; staining and culture of pus aspirated from brain abscess confirm polymicrobial infection.

Imaging CT (with contrast): multiple ring-enhancing lesions with low attenuation centers (ABSCESS) surrounding cerebral edema and ventricular compression.

Gross Pathology Cavity filled with thick, liquefied pus surrounded by fibrous capsule of variable thickness; pericapsular zone of gliosis and edema.

Micro Pathology Central portion contains degenerated PMNs and cellular debris; capsule is composed of collagenous fibrous tissue with blood vessels and mixed inflammatory cells.

Treatment High-dose, extended parenteral broad-spectrum antibiotic coverage; **CT-directed drainage of pus.**

Discussion Brain abscesses arise secondary to **hematogenous spread** from another infection (bronchiectasis, endocarditis), from contiguous spread from adjacent infection (chronic otitis media, mastoiditis, sinusitis), or following **direct implantation** from trauma. Patients with congenital heart disease with right-to-left shunt are particularly predisposed because the normal filtering action of the pulmonary vasculature is lost.

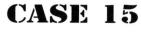

CASE 15

ID/CC

A 25-year-old puerpera who was **lactating** her week-old infant presents with **pain and swelling** in her left breast.

HPI

The symptoms commenced acutely, and she does not recall any previous breast lumps or swellings.

PE

Skin overlying left breast is **red, edematous, tender, and hot**; area of tense induration felt underlying inflamed skin.

Labs

Culture of pus drained from **breast abscess** and **nasopharyngeal swab** taken from the infant **grew** *Staphylococcus aureus*.

Imaging

USG: nearly anechoic area with posterior enhancement.

Treatment

Penicillinase-resistant antibiotic; incision (in a radial direction over the affected segment) **and dependent drainage** of intramammary abscess; patient may continue nursing from the affected breast.

Discussion

Bacterial mastitis most commonly occurs in lactating women due to infection of a hematoma or secondary infection of plasma cell mastitis; the infecting **organism is mostly penicillin-resistant** *Staphylococcus aureus*.

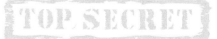

ID/CC   A 28-year-old white male visits his family doctor complaining of acute **pain in both hip joints** together with weakness, backache, myalgias, arthralgias, and **undulating fever** of **2 months'** duration; this morning he woke up with pain in his right testicle.

HPI   For the past 3 years he has worked at the largest dairy farm in his state. He enjoys **drinking "crude" milk.**

PE   VS: fever. PE: pallor; marked pain on palpation of sacroiliac joints; mild splenomegaly; generalized lymphadenopathy.

Labs   CBC: relative lymphocytosis with normal WBC count. Positive agglutination titer (> 1:160); rising serologic titer over time; small gram-negative rod *Brucella abortus* on blood culture.

Imaging   XR, hips: joint effusion and soft tissue swelling without destruction. MR, spine: evidence of spondylitis.

Gross Pathology   Lymphadenopathy and splenomegaly; hepatomegaly rare.

Micro Pathology   Granulomatous foci in spleen, liver, and lymph nodes, with proliferation of macrophages; epithelioid and giant cells may be seen.

Treatment   Combination therapy with doxycycline or TMP-SMX and rifampin or streptomycin.

Discussion   Also called Malta fever, a microbial disease of animals, brucellosis is caused by several species of *Brucella*, a gram-negative, aerobic coccobacillus. It is transmitted to humans through the drinking of contaminated milk or through direct contact with products or tissues from animals such as goats, sheep, camels, cows, hogs, and dogs. The clinical picture is often vague; thus, a high index of suspicion may be necessary for diagnosis.

ID/CC	A 26-year-old female presents to the ER with intense, acute-onset left **lower quadrant crampy abdominal pain,** foul-smelling stools with streaks of blood, urgency, **tenesmus,** and fever.
HPI	For the past 2 days, the patient has also had headaches and myalgias. She frequently **drinks unpasteurized** ("raw") **milk** that she buys at a health-food store.
PE	VS: fever (39°C); tachycardia; normal RR and BP. PE: no dehydration; diffuse abdominal tenderness more marked in left lower quadrant.
Labs	Stool smear shows leukocytes (due to invasive tissue damage in the colon) and **gram-negative, curved bacilli,** often in pairs, in "gull-wing"-shaped pattern; dark-field exam shows motility; culture in micro-aerophilic, 42°C conditions on special agar yields *Campylobacter jejuni,* indicated by oxidase and catalase positivity.
Gross Pathology	Friable colonic mucosa.
Micro Pathology	Nonspecific inflammatory reaction consisting of neutrophils, lympho-cytes and plasma cells with hyperemia, edema and damage to epithelium, glandular degeneration, ulcerations, and crypt abscesses caused by colonic tissue invasion of the organism.
Treatment	Fluid and electrolyte replacement; macrolides (e.g., erythromycin) for persistent or severe disease.
Discussion	One of the primary causes of "traveler's diarrhea." Sources of infection include **undercooked food** and contact with **infected animals** and their excreta. Prevent by improving public sanitation, pasteurizing milk, and proper cooking.

TOP SECRET

ID/CC   A 25-year-old female presents with **painful lumps in her right axilla** and neck together with **low-grade fever**.

HPI   Three weeks ago she was **scratched** on her right forearm **by her pet cat**; an erythematous pustule initially developed at the site but resolved spontaneously within 10 days.

PE   VS: fever. PE: **tender right axillary** and cervical **lymphadenopathy**.

Labs   Lymph node biopsy diagnostic; serologic indirect immunofluorescent antibody test for *Bartonella henselae* is positive.

Micro Pathology   Hematoxylin and eosin staining reveals **granulomatous pathology** with stellate necrosis and surrounding palisades of histiocytic cells; **Warthin–Starry silver stain** reveals **clumps of pleomorphic, strongly argyrophilic bacilli**.

Treatment   Disease is usually self-limited in immunocompetent hosts; immunocompromised patients may need antibiotic treatment with rifampin, ciprofloxacin, TMP-SMX, or gentamicin.

Discussion   *Bartonella henselae* is the agent that causes cat-scratch disease. Lymphadenopathy can persist for months and can sometimes be mistaken for a malignancy. Individuals who are immunocompromised may present with seizures, coma, and meningitis.

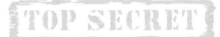

CASE 19

ID/CC

A 54-year-old female who **underwent** a left mastectomy with **axillary lymph node dissection** a year ago presents with **pain** together with rapidly spreading **redness** and **swelling** of the left **arm**.

HPI

One year ago, she was diagnosed and operated on for stage 1 **carcinoma of the left breast.**

PE

Left forearm swollen, indurated, pink, and markedly tender; overlying temperature raised; margins and borders of skin lesion ill defined and not elevated (vs. erysipelas).

Labs

Needle aspiration from advancing border of the lesion, when stained and cultured, isolated β-hemolytic group A streptococcus.

Treatment

Penicillinase-resistant penicillin (nafcillin/oxacillin).

Discussion

Cellulitis is an acute spreading infection of the skin that predominantly affects deeper subcutaneous tissue. **Group A streptococci and** *Staphylococcus aureus* are the **most common** etiologic agents in adults; *Haemophilus influenzae* infection is common in children. Patients with chronic venous stasis and lymphedema of any cause (lymphoma, filariasis, post–regional lymph node dissection, radiation therapy) are predisposed; recently, recurrent saphenous-vein donor-site cellulitis was found to be attributable to group A, C, or G streptococci.

ID/CC   A 35-year-old male complains of **cough** productive of mucopurulent sputum and **breathlessness**.

HPI   Before the onset of these symptoms, he had a sore throat with hoarseness. He has no history of hemoptysis, sharp chest pain, or high-grade fever.

PE   Crepitations heard over left lung base.

Labs   CBC: normal leukocyte count. Sputum exam revealed no **bacterial organism**; positive indirect microimmunofluorescence test for *Chlamydia pneumoniae* antibodies; cultivation of *C. pneumoniae* demonstrated on HL cell line.

Imaging   CXR: left lower lobe subsegmental infiltrate with interstitial pattern.

Treatment **Doxycycline** is the drug of choice; alternatively, **erythromycin** may be used.

Discussion *Chlamydia pneumoniae* causes mild lower respiratory infection in young adults, but older adults suffer more serious disease. It is transmitted by respiratory droplets.

TOP SECRET

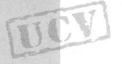

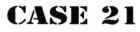

CASE 21

ID/CC An 8-year-old male who recently emigrated from India presents with **bilateral eye irritation** and **photophobia**.

HPI He reports **recurrent episodes** of similar eye irritation and redness **in the past**.

PE Conjunctival congestion; **multiple (> 5) follicles**, each at least 0.5 mm in diameter, seen **in upper tarsal conjunctiva**; inflammatory thickening of tarsal conjunctiva; new vessels (PANNUS) seen in cornea at superior limbus; **punctate keratitis**.

Labs Cell culture grows *Chlamydia trachomatis*; positive direct immunofluorescence for **elementary bodies**.

Micro Pathology *C. trachomatis* is typically seen in conjunctival scrapings in colony form in the epithelial cells as H-P inclusion bodies. Histologically there is lymphocytic infiltration involving the whole adenoid layer of parts of the conjunctiva; special aggregations of lymphocytes form **follicles** that tend to show necrosis and certain large multinucleated cells (LEBER'S CELLS).

Treatment Topical **tetracycline** or erythromycin with systemic **tetracycline/doxycycline/erythromycin** for possible extraocular infection (GI or nasopharyngeal); prophylaxis of family contacts with topical tetracycline.

Discussion *Chlamydia trachomatis* causes a variety of ocular diseases, including **neonatal inclusion conjunctivitis, sporadic inclusion conjunctivitis in adults, and sporadic as well as endemic trachoma**; trachoma is endemic in North Africa, in the Middle East, and among the Native American population of the southwestern United States. In endemic areas, trachoma is transmitted from eye to hand to eye, especially among young children in regions where standards of cleanliness are poor. Sporadic trachoma infection in nonendemic areas as well as sporadic inclusion conjunctivitis in adults results from transmission of the agent from the genital tract to the eye. Trachoma is a **major cause of blindness** in endemic areas.

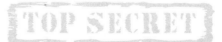

ID/CC   A 30-year-old man has sudden severe, **profuse (several liters per day) watery diarrhea, protracted vomiting,** and **abdominal pain.**

HPI   He has just returned from a trip to **rural India.**

PE   **Severe dehydration;** low urine output; generalized mild abdominal tenderness with no signs of peritoneal irritation; stools have characteristic **"rice-water" appearance** (gray, slightly cloudy fluid with flecks of mucus), with no blood.

Labs   Stool culture reveals gram-negative rods with **"darting motility";** O1 **antigen detected;** *Vibrio cholerae* isolated on culture media; serum chloride levels decreased; serum sodium levels increased.

Treatment   **Vigorous rehydration** therapy with oral and/or IV fluids; **tetracycline,** ciprofloxacin, or doxycycline.

Discussion   A heat-labile exotoxin produced by *Vibrio cholerae* that acts by permanently **stimulating G_s protein via ADP ribosylation,** resulting in activation of **intracellular adenylate cyclase,** which in turn increases cAMP levels and produces **secretory diarrhea.**

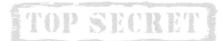

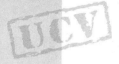

ID/CC   A 28-year-old primigravida at 36 weeks' gestation presents with a **high fever**.

HPI   She was being monitored following a **premature rupture of the membranes**.

PE   VS: **fever**; fetal tachycardia. PE: **uterine tenderness**.

Labs   Elevated maternal total lymphocyte count; **vaginal swab** culture revealed colonization with **group B streptococcus**.

Treatment   Presence of group B streptococcus in vagina after premature rupture of membranes was an indication for **immediate delivery and treatment of the infant**; mother was also treated with an **antibiotic** regimen that included clindamycin, gentamicin, and ampicillin.

Discussion   A significant proportion of the population is colonized in the vagina and rectum with **group B streptococcus, which is correlated with preterm labor, premature rupture of membranes** (PROM), **chorioamnionitis, and neonatal sepsis**; neonates with group B streptococcus sepsis have a 25% mortality rate. Among preterm neonates, this figure doubles to over 50%; therefore **antibiotic prophylaxis** is recommended in the setting of **preterm delivery and PROM** even without the diagnosis of frank chorioamnionitis. When chorioamnionitis is suspected, intravenous antibiotics are started and delivery is hastened.

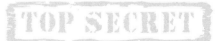

ID/CC	A **5-year-old** white male presents with malaise, anorexia, low-grade fever, sore throat of 3 days' duration, and dyspnea on exertion.
HPI	The child was raised abroad. His immunization status cannot be determined.
PE	VS: fever; tachycardia with occasional dropped beats. PE: **cervical lymphadenopathy** (BULL'S-NECK APPEARANCE); smooth, **whitish-gray, adherent membrane over tonsils and pharynx**; no hepatosplenomegaly; diminished intensity of S1.
Labs	**Metachromatic granules** in **bacilli arranged in "Chinese character" pattern** on Albert stain of throat culture; *Corynebacterium diphtheriae* confirmed by growth observed on **Löffler's blood agar**; erythema and necrosis following intradermal injection of *C. diphtheriae* toxin (POSITIVE SCHICK'S TEST); immunodiffusion studies (Elek's) confirm toxigenic strains of *C. diphtheriae*. ECG: ST-segment elevation; second-degree heart block.
Imaging	Echo: evidence of myocarditis.
Gross Pathology	Pharyngeal membranes not restricted to anatomic landmarks; pale and enlarged heart.
Micro Pathology	Polymorphonuclear exudate with bacteria; precipitated fibrin and cell debris forming a **pseudomembrane**; marked hyperemia, edema, and necrosis of upper respiratory tract mucosa; exotoxin-induced myofibrillar hyaline degeneration; lysis of myelin sheath.
Treatment	Begin treatment on presumptive diagnosis; specific antitoxin and penicillin or erythromycin; respiratory and cardiac support; confirm eradication by repeating throat culture.
Discussion	A bacterial infection of the throat, diphtheria is preventable by vaccine and is caused by toxigenic *Corynebacterium diphtheriae*, a club-shaped, gram-positive aerobic bacillus. Diphtheria toxin is produced by β-prophage-infected corynebacteria; it blocks EF-2 via ADP ribosylation and hence ribosomal function in protein synthesis. The toxin enters the bloodstream, causing **fever, myocarditis** (within the first 2 weeks), and **polyneuritis** (many weeks later).

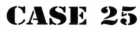

CASE 25

ID/CC A 28-year-old male who is a resident of the **southeastern United States** presents with a high **fever with chills, headache, and myalgias.**

HPI He remembers having been **bitten by a tick** a week before developing his symptoms; however, he reports no skin rash.

PE VS: fever. PE: no skin rash noted.

Labs CBC: leukopenia and mild thrombocytopenia. **Characteristic intra-leukocytic inclusion bodies** (MORULAE) and serologic response to *Ehrlichia* antigens demonstrated; *E. chaffeensis* cultured from blood and detected by PCR.

Treatment Doxycycline.

Discussion Ehrlichieae are gram-negative, obligately intracellular bacteria. The two types of *Ehrlichia* species that affect humans are *E. chaffeensis* (which attacks macrophages and monocytes) and an *E. equi*-like organism (which attacks granulocytes). Preventive measures include wearing clothing that covers the body and using insect repellants.

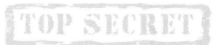

ID/CC   A 30-year-old male from **Texas** presents with **fever and a skin rash** that began about 2 weeks ago.

HPI   The onset was gradual, with prodromal symptoms of headache, malaise, backache, and chills. These symptoms were followed by shaking chills, fever, and a more severe headache accompanied by nausea and vomiting. A remittent pattern of fever accompanied by tachycardia continued for 10 to 12 days, with the **rash appearing around the fifth day of fever**. The patient **worked at a rat-infested food-storage depot** this summer.

PE   VS: fever. PE: discrete, irregular pink **maculopapular rash** seen in axillae and on trunk, thighs, and upper arms; face, palms, and soles only sparsely involved; mild splenomegaly noted.

Labs   The **Weil–Felix** agglutination reaction for *Proteus* strain **OX-19 was positive**; complement-fixing antibodies to the typhus group antigen were demonstrated; **endemic typhus** (due to *Rickettsia typhi*) **was confirmed serologically** by using specific washed rickettsial antigens in IFA tests.

Treatment   Antibiotic treatment with **doxycycline** (**chloramphenicol** is used as an alternative).

Discussion   Murine typhus is a natural infection of rats and mice by *Rickettsia typhi*; **spread of infection to humans by the rat flea** is incidental and occurs when feces from infected fleas are scratched into the lesion. Cases can occur year-round; however, most occur during the summer months, primarily in southern Texas and California.

TOP SECRET

ID/CC A 28-year-old Guatemalan male is brought to the hospital complaining of **severe headache**, photophobia, and fever over the past 2 weeks.

HPI As a political dissident, he spent 4 months in a **refugee camp** in southern Mexico before entering the United States.

PE VS: fever (40°C). PE: papilledema and delirium; bilateral swelling of parotid glands 1 week later; toxic facies; maculopapular **rash** on trunk and extremities; **face, palms, and soles spared**; mild splenomegaly.

Labs **Positive Weil-Felix reaction** to OX-19 strains of *Proteus*; rise in complement fixation titer for *Rickettsia prowazekii*; specific antibodies. UA: proteinuria; microscopic hematuria.

Gross Pathology Myocarditis and pneumonia may be present; cerebral edema; maculopapular rash.

Micro Pathology **Zenker's degeneration of striated muscle**; thrombosis and endothelial proliferation of capillaries with abundant rickettsiae and perivascular cuffing; accumulation of lymphocytes; microglia and macrophages **(typhus nodules)** in brain.

Treatment **Doxycycline**; chloramphenicol.

Discussion Epidemic typhus is a febrile illness caused by *Rickettsia prowazekii*, a gram-negative, nonmotile, obligate intracellular parasite; it is transmitted via **body lice** and is associated with **war, famine,** and **crowded living conditions**. The rash should be differentiated from Rocky Mountain spotted fever, which starts peripherally on the wrists and ankles and also includes the palms and soles.

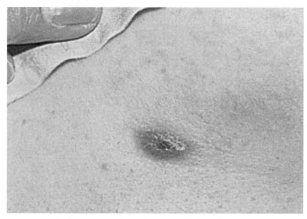

Figure 027 Erythematous macule with central black eschar.

ID/CC   A **28-year-old man** comes to the ER with gradually worsening and now severe **scrotal swelling** and pain radiating to the inguinal area.

HPI   The patient has no significant medical history. He reports pain on urination (due to concomitant urethritis) and notes that he is sexually active with multiple partners. He also notes that the pain is greater on standing and walking and is relieved by rest and elevation of the legs.

PE   VS: normal. PE: **scrotal edema** and erythema; **right epididymis enlarged and tender**; induration present; **elevation** of scrotal contents **relieves pain** (PREHN'S SIGN).

Labs   UA: pyuria. Culture negative; biopsy of epididymis inoculated into cell cultures grows *Chlamydia trachomatis*; immunofluorescence reveals **subtype D**.

Imaging   US: hypoechoic, enlarged epididymis with hypervascularity.

Gross Pathology   Nonspecific inflammation characterized by congestion and edema.

Micro Pathology   Early stage of the infection is limited to the interstitial connective tissue with white cell infiltration.

Treatment   Antibiotics like doxycycline, minocycline for chlamydia. Course of ofloxacin covers all possibilities of causative organisms.

Discussion   Differentiate epididymitis from testicular torsion and tumor (scrotal ultrasonography or isotopic flow study may be needed for differentiating). Transmitted sexually in young adults and most often **caused by *Chlamydia trachomatis* subtypes D through K** and *Neisseria gonorrhoeae*. In those older than 40, *Escherichia coli* and *Pseudomonas* cause most infections. If associated with rectal intercourse, it may be due to Enterobacteriaceae.

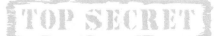

ID/CC   A **4-year-old** male presents with **fever, hoarseness,** and respiratory distress because of partial **airway obstruction.**

HPI   The child is also **unable to speak clearly and has pain while swallowing** (ODYNOPHAGIA).

PE   VS: fever; tachypnea. PE: **patient is leaning forward with neck hyperextended and chin protruding; drooling;** marked suprasternal and infrasternal retraction of chest; **inspiratory stridor** on auscultation.

Labs   Culture of throat swab (no role in management of acute disease) reveals penicillinase-resistant *Haemophilus influenzae*; blood cultures also positive.

Imaging   XR, neck: marked edema of epiglottis and aryepiglottic folds ("THUMBS-UP" SIGN).

Gross Pathology   Epiglottis is cherry-red, swollen, and "angry-looking." Rapid cellulitis of epiglottis and surrounding tissue leads to progressive blockage of airway.

Treatment   Preservation of airway; IV cefuroxime; rifampin prophylaxis for contacts.

Discussion   The principal cause of acute epiglottitis in children and adults is *H. influenzae* type b; other pathogens include *H. parainfluenzae* and group A streptococcus. Characterized by rapid onset.

ID/CC

A 16-year-old teenager presents to the outpatient clinic with a **painful facial rash** and **fever**.

HPI

One week ago, the patient went on a camping trip and scratched his face on some low-lying tree branches. There is no medical history of diabetes, cancer, or other chronic conditions.

PE

VS: **fever** (39.0°C); **tachycardia** (HR 110); BP normal. PE: **erythematous, warm, plaque-like rash** extending across cheeks and face bilaterally with **sharp, distinct borders** and **facial swelling**.

Labs

CBC: **leukocytosis** with **neutrophilia. ESR elevated.**

Treatment

Antibiotics with sufficient coverage for penicillinase-producing *Streptococcus* and *Staphylococcus* spp. (e.g., cephalexin); **analgesics/ antipyretics**; elevate the affected part to reduce swelling.

Discussion

Erysipelas is an acute inflammation of the superficial layers of the connective tissues of the skin, usually on the face, almost always caused by infection with group A streptococcus, which is part of normal bacterial skin flora. Risk factors include any breaks in the skin or **lymphedema**.

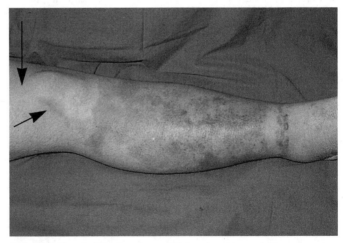

Figure 030 Sharply defined erythema with lymphangitic streak (arrows).

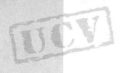

CASE 31

ID/CC

A 30-year-old **slaughterhouse worker** presents with a **painful red swelling** of the **index finger** of his right hand.

HPI

The swelling developed 4 days after he was **injured** with a knife **while slaughtering a pig**.

PE

Well-defined, exquisitely tender, slightly elevated **violaceous lesion seen on right index finger**; no suppuration noted; right epitrochlear and right axillary lymphadenopathy noted.

Labs

Biopsy from edge of lesion yields *Erysipelothrix rhusiopathiae*, a thin, pleomorphic, nonsporulating, microaerophilic gram-positive rod.

Treatment

Penicillin G: erythromycin and rifampin for patients allergic to penicillin.

Discussion

Erysipeloid refers to **localized cellulitis**, usually of the fingers and hands, caused by *Erysipelothrix rhusiopathiae*; infection in humans is usually the result of **contact with infected animals** or their products (**often fish**). Organisms gain entry via cuts and abrasions on the skin.

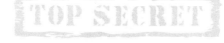

ID/CC	A 30-year-old female presents to the surgical ER complaining of a stabbing **right upper quadrant abdominal pain.**
HPI	She is a prostitute who has been receiving treatment for **gonococcal pelvic inflammatory disease.**
PE	Right upper quadrant tenderness; cervical motion tenderness and mucopurulent cervicitis found on pelvic exam.
Labs	Cervical swab staining and culture identifies *Neisseria gonorrhoeae.*
Imaging	US: no evidence of cholecystitis. Peritoneoscopy: presence of "violin string" **adhesions between liver capsule and peritoneum.**
Gross Pathology	Adhesions noted between liver capsule and peritoneum.
Treatment	Antibiotic therapy (ceftriaxone and doxycycline) for patient (and for partner if warranted).
Discussion	**Acute fibrinous perihepatitis** (FITZ–HUGH–CURTIS SYNDROME) occurs as a complication of **gonococcal and chlamydial pelvic inflammatory disease** and clinically mimics cholecystitis.

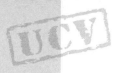

CASE 33

ID/CC
A 30-year-old soldier who had been admitted for a **gunshot wound** in the right thigh presents with **severe pain and swelling** at the site of his injury.

HPI
The patient's right lower limb had become discolored, and several bullae had appeared on the skin. He has passed very little urine over the past day, and the urine he has passed has been dark ("cola-colored").

PE
VS: low-grade fever; marked tachycardia. PE: diaphoresis; skin of right thigh discolored (bronze to purple red); site of injury exquisitely tender and tense and **oozing** a thin, dark, and **foul-smelling fluid**; **crepitus** while palpating thigh.

Labs
CBC: low hematocrit. Gram stain of exudate and necrotic material at wound site reveals presence of **large gram-positive rods**; anaerobic culture of exudate and blood yields *Clostridium perfringens* type A; culture isolate demonstrates **positive Nagler reaction** (due to presence of alpha toxin lecithinase); further labs confirm presence of **intravascular hemolysis, myo- and hemoglobinuria**, and **acute tubular necrosis**.

Imaging
XR, right thigh: presence of **gas in soft tissues**.

Gross Pathology
Overlying skin purple-bronze, markedly edematous with vesiculobullous changes with little suppurative reaction.

Micro Pathology
Coagulative necrosis, edema, **gas formation**, and many large **gram-positive bacilli** found in affected muscle tissue; relatively sparse infiltration of PMNs noted in the bordering muscle tissue.

Treatment
Surgical debridement; antibiotics (penicillin, clindamycin, tetracycline, metronidazole); hyperbaric oxygen therapy and polyvalent antitoxin; supportive management of associated multiorgan failure.

Discussion
A rapidly progressive myonecrosis caused by *Clostridium perfringens* type A, traumatic gas gangrene develops in a wound with low oxygen tension (embedded foreign bodies containing calcium or silicates cause lowering of oxygen tension, leading to germination of the spores). The most important toxin is the alpha toxin lecithinase, which produces hemolysis and myonecrosis.

ID/CC   A 25-year-old male presents with sudden-onset, severe **vomiting**, nausea, **abdominal cramps, and diarrhea**.

HPI   He had returned home about 2 hours after attending a birthday party at which **meat and milk** were served in various forms. The **friend** who was celebrating his birthday **reported similar symptoms**.

PE   VS: **no fever**. PE: mild dehydration; diffuse abdominal tenderness; increased bowel sounds.

Labs   **Toxigenic staphylococcus** recovered from culturing food. Coagulase-positive staphylococcus cultured from **nose of one of the cooks** at party.

Micro Pathology   No mucosal lesions.

Treatment   Fluid and electrolyte balance; antibiotics not indicated.

Discussion   *Staphylococcus aureus* food poisoning results from the ingestion of food containing **preformed heat-stable enterotoxin B**. Outbreaks of staphylococcal food poisoning occur when **food handlers** who have contaminated superficial wounds or who are shedding infected nasal droplets inoculate foods such as meat, dairy products, salad dressings, cream sauces, and custard-filled pastries. The **incubation period** ranges from **2 to 8 hours**; the disease is self-limited.

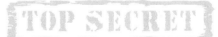

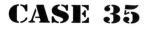

ID/CC A **3-day-old** female neonate presents with a **thick eye discharge**.

HPI The **mother** admits to having **multiple sexual partners** and complains of a **vaginal discharge**. She did not receive adequate antenatal care.

PE Exam of both eyes reveals a **thick purulent discharge** and marked **conjunctival congestion** and edema; conjunctival **chemosis** is so marked that cornea is seen at bottom of a crater-like pit; **corneal ulceration** noted.

Labs Conjunctival swabs on Gram staining reveal presence of **gram-negative diplococci** both intra- and extracellularly in addition to **many PMNs**; conjunctival swab and maternal cervical culture yield *Neisseria gonorrhoeae*.

Treatment **Penicillin G** or **ceftriaxone**. Also treat mother and her sexual contacts.

Discussion Caused by *Neisseria gonorrhoeae*, gonococcal ophthalmia neonatorum is **contracted** from a mother with gonorrhea **as the fetus passes down the birth canal**; infection does not occur in utero. **Corneal inflammation** is the major clinical sign that may produce complications such as corneal opacities, perforation, anterior synechiae, anterior staphyloma, and panophthalmitis. It is now common practice to **prevent** this disease by treating the **eyes of the newborn with an antibacterial** compound such as erythromycin ointment or 1% silver nitrate; however, home childbirth bypasses this prophylactic procedure, and thus some cases are still occurring in the United States.

TOP SECRET

ID/CC   A 19-year-old white male presents with **burning urination**; profuse, **greenish-yellow, purulent urethral discharge**; staining of his underwear; and urethral pain.

HPI   Four days ago, he had **unprotected sexual contact** with a prostitute.

PE   **Mucopurulent** and slightly blood-tinged urethral discharge; normal testes and epididymis; no urinary retention.

Labs   Smear of urethral discharge reveals **intracellular gram-negative diplococci** in WBCs; gonococcal infection confirmed by inoculation into **Thayer-Martin medium**.

Gross Pathology   Abundant, purulent urethral exudate.

Treatment   Ceftriaxone; add doxycycline or erythromycin for **possible coinfection with *Chlamydia***.

Discussion   A common STD caused by *Neisseria gonorrhoeae*, gonorrhea may involve the throat, anus, rectum, epididymis, cervix, fallopian tubes, prostate, and joints; conjunctivitis is also found in neonates. Neonatal conjunctivitis may be prevented through the instillation of silver nitrate or erythromycin eye drops at birth.

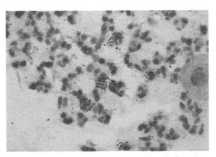

Figure 036A Gram-negative diplococci in a urethral specimen.

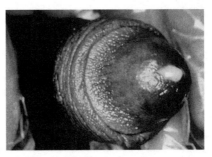

Figure 036B Purulent urethral discharge.

CASE 37

ID/CC

A 45-year-old male with refractory **acute myeloid leukemia** who underwent a **bone marrow transplant** from a nonidentical donor presents with an **extensive skin rash**, severe **diarrhea**, and **jaundice**.

HPI

Prior to the transplant, which occurred 2 months ago, he **received preparative chemotherapy and radiotherapy** along with broad-spectrum antibiotics. Engraftment was confirmed within 4 weeks by rising leukocyte counts.

PE

VS: BP normal. PE: patient is cachectic and moderately dehydrated; icterus noted; violaceous, scaly macules and erythematous papules **resembling lichen planus** seen over extremities.

Labs

CBC: falling blood counts; relative eosinophilia. Elevated direct serum bilirubin and transaminases; stool exam reveals no infectious etiology; skin biopsy taken.

Gross Pathology

Skin biopsy specimens reveal vacuolar changes of basal cell layer with perivenular lymphocytic infiltrates (CD8+ T cells).

Treatment

High-dose cyclosporine therapy, anti-thymocyte globulin, methylprednisolone or anti-T-cell monoclonal antibodies.

Discussion

Approximately 30% of bone marrow transplant recipients develop graft-versus-host disease (GVHD). This attack is primarily launched by immunocompetent T lymphocytes derived from the donor's marrow against the cells and tissues of the recipient, which it recognizes as foreign. Cyclosporin A is effective for prevention of GVHD.

ID/CC	A 28-year-old male **immigrant** presents with **inguinal swelling** and a **painless penile ulcer.**
HPI	He admits to unprotected intercourse with **multiple sexual partners,** many of whom were prostitutes. He first noticed a papule on his penis several weeks ago.
PE	Soft, **painless,** raised, **beefy-red,** smooth **granulating ulcer** noted on distal penis; multiple **subcutaneous swellings** (PSEUDOBUBOES) noted in inguinal region, some of which have ulcerated.
Labs	Giemsa-stained smear from penile and inguinal regions demonstrate characteristic "**closed safety pin**" appearance of encapsulated organisms **within a large histiocyte** (DONOVAN BODIES).
Micro Pathology	Characteristic histologic picture of donovanosis comprises some degree of epithelial hyperplasia at margins of lesions; dense plasma cell infiltrate scatters histiocyte-containing Donovan bodies.
Treatment	Treat with **doxycycline** or **TMP-SMX.**
Discussion	Granuloma inguinale, a slowly progressive, ulcerative, granulomatous STD involving the genitalia, is caused by the gram-negative bacillus *Calymmatobacterium granulomatis* (formerly *Donovania granulomatis*); it is seen in Giemsa-stained sections as a dark-staining, encapsulated, intra-cellular rod-shaped inclusion in macrophages, the so-called **Donovan body.** The disease is endemic in tropical areas such as New Guinea, southern India, and southern Africa.

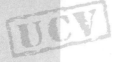

ID/CC

A 60-year-old **male** presents with **cough productive of mucopurulent sputum** together with mild fever and worsening breathlessness.

HPI

He is a chronic smoker who has been diagnosed with COPD.

PE

VS: fever. PE: in moderate respiratory distress; emphysematous chest with obliterated cardiac and liver dullness; **wheezing and crackles** heard over both lung fields.

Labs

Haemophilus influenzae organisms seen as small, pleomorphic gram-negative bacilli on Gram stain of sputum; **nontypable *H. influenzae* isolated on sputum culture** (to grow in culture, *H. influenzae* requires both factor X–hematin and factor V–nicotinamide nucleoside present in erythrocytes).

Treatment

Amoxicillin/ampicillin therapy; alternatively, TMP-SMX, azithromycin, or cefuroxime.

Discussion

Infections caused by nontypable, or unencapsulated, *Haemophilus influenzae* strains have been increasingly recognized in pediatric and adult populations. Nontypable *H. influenzae* strains are frequent respiratory tract colonizers in patients with COPD and commonly exacerbate chronic bronchitis in these patients; nontypable strains are also the most common cause of acute otitis media in children.

TOP SECRET

ID/CC   A 20-year-old male presents with an extensive **purpuric skin rash, oliguria**, and marked weakness; he also complains of **bloody diarrhea** of 1 week's duration.

HPI   The patient ate **a hamburger** at a fast-food restaurant 2 to 3 **days prior to the onset** of his diarrhea. He has no associated fever.

PE   VS: no fever. PE: dehydration; pallor; extensive purpuric skin rash.

Labs   Stool examination reveals presence of RBCs but **no inflammatory cells** or parasites; culture isolates sorbitol-negative *Escherichia coli*; serotyping studies and effect on HeLa cell culture reveal presence of **enterohemorrhagic *E. coli* (EHEC) serotype O157:H7**; elevated BUN and creatinine. CBC/PBS: **microangiopathic anemia** and thrombocytopenia. PT, PTT normal.

Imaging   Sigmoidoscopy: moderately hyperemic mucosa with no evidence of any ulceration.

Micro Pathology   Pathology localized to kidney, where hyaline **thrombi** were seen **in afferent arterioles** and glomerular capillaries.

Treatment   Dialysis and blood transfusion for management of HUS; fluid and electrolyte maintenance; antimicrobial therapy. Most patients who develop HUS as a complication of *E. coli* hemorrhagic colitis die as a result of hemorrhagic complications.

Discussion   Hemorrhagic colitis associated with a Shiga-like toxin producing EHEC O157:H7 is characterized by grossly bloody diarrhea with remarkably little fever or inflammatory exudate in stool; a significant number of patients develop potentially fatal HUS. EHEC infections can be largely **prevented through adequate cooking of beef**, especially hamburgers.

ID/CC   A 5-year-old white male presents with golden-yellow, crusted lesions around his mouth and behind his ears.

HPI   He has a history of intermittent low-grade fever, frequent "nose picking," and purulent discharge from his lesions. He has no history of hematuria (due to increased risk of poststreptococcal glomerulonephritis).

PE   Characteristic "honey-colored" crusted lesions seen at angle of mouth, around nasal orifices, and behind ears.

Labs   Gram-positive cocci in chains (STREPTOCOCCI) in addition to pus cells on Gram stain of discharge; β-hemolytic streptococci (group A streptococci) on blood agar culture; ASO titer negative.

Gross Pathology   Erythematous lesions surrounding natural orifices with whitish or yellowish purulent exudate and crust formation.

Micro Pathology   Inflammatory infiltrate of PMNs with varying degrees of necrosis.

Treatment Cephalosporin, penicillin, or erythromycin if allergic.

Discussion Impetigo is a highly communicable infectious disease that is most often caused by group A streptococci, occurs primarily in preschoolers, and may predispose to glomerulonephritis. It occurs most commonly on the face (periorbital area), hands, and arms. *Staphylococcus aureus* may coexist or cause bullous impetigo; group B streptococcal impetigo may be seen in newborns.

ID/CC	A **2-day-old** neonate is evaluated for an **eye discharge**.
HPI	The baby's **mother is a prostitute** who did not receive any prenatal cervical cultures during pregnancy.
PE	Normal full-term male neonate; mucoid **eye discharge, conjunctival congestion, and chemosis** noted in both eyes; nonfollicles seen on palpebral conjunctiva (due to absence of subconjunctival adenoid layer at this age); mild **superficial keratitis** also present.
Labs	Gram stain of swab reveals increased **PMNs** and **no bacteria**; characteristic **intracellular inclusion bodies demonstrated by the DIF test**; cell culture yields *Chlamydia trachomatis* **serotypes D through K**; chlamydia also grown from **maternal cervical swab**.
Treatment	Oral **erythromycin**; no topical therapy; also treat mother and her partners.
Discussion	*Chlamydia trachomatis* is an important cause of preventable blindness; its strains can be further differentiated into 18 serotypes by microimmunofluorescence tests. **Serotypes A, B, Ba, and C** are principally associated with **endemic trachoma** in developing countries; **serotypes D through K** primarily cause **sexually transmitted** infections in adults and **inclusion conjunctivitis and pneumonia in infants**, transmitted through an infected birth canal; and **serotypes L1, L2, and L3** cause **lymphogranuloma venereum**.

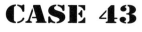

ID/CC

A 30-year-old female presents with **fever, chills**, malaise, headaches, and **myalgias**.

HPI

She was diagnosed as suffering from **secondary syphilis** with an extensive nonpruritic **skin rash, condylomata lata**, and **mucous patches** in the mouth, for which she received a dose of intramuscular **penicillin 6 hours ago**.

PE

VS: **fever**; tachycardia; mild hypotension.

Treatment

No specific treatment; symptoms subside in 24 hours.

Discussion

The Jarisch-Herxheimer reaction consists of fever, chills, mild hypotension, headache, and an increase in the intensity of mucocutaneous lesions **2 hours after** initiating **treatment of syphilis with penicillin** or another effective antibiotic; symptoms usually **subside in 12 to 24 hours**. The reaction occurs in 50% of patients with primary syphilis and in 90% of those with secondary syphilis. The Jarisch-Herxheimer reaction **also occurs after treatment of other spirochetal diseases** (e.g., louse-borne relapsing fever caused by *Borrelia recurrentis*). It has been suggested that the release of treponemal lipopolysaccharides might produce this symptom complex.

ID/CC	A 40-year-old male smoker complains of acute-onset **high fever**, chills, a **nonproductive cough**, tachypnea, and **pleuritic chest pain**.
HPI	A number of **similar cases** have been reported in his workplace in recent months. The patient admits to significant alcohol and tobacco consumption and uses a **humidifier** at night.
PE	VS: fever; dyspnea. PE: rales present bilaterally on auscultation.
Labs	Sputum exam with Gram stain reveals no pathogenic organisms. CBC: neutrophilic leukocytosis. Urine ELISA positive for *Legionella* antigen; sputum culture isolates *Legionella*; cold agglutinins absent; indirect fluorescent antibody technique reveals stable titer of > 1:256 (considered diagnostic); **direct immunofluorescent** staining of sputum confirms presence of *Legionella*.
Imaging	CXR, PA: bilateral diffuse, patchy infiltrates and **ill-defined nodules**.
Gross Pathology	Nodular areas of consolidation that may progress to involvement of one or more lobes of the lung.
Micro Pathology	Alveolar exudate with PMNs, macrophages, and fibrin; in more severe cases, destruction of alveolar septa.
Treatment	Fluoroquinolone or macrolide therapy.
Discussion	Legionnaire's disease is caused by *Legionella pneumophila*, a filamentous, flagellated, aerobic gram-negative, motile bacillus, and is more common in immunocompromised patients. Epidemiologic studies have established **drinking water** and **air conditioners** as the sources of outbreak.

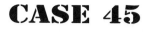

ID/CC

A 30-year-old male from **India** presents with slowly progressive **hypopigmented skin patches and nodules** together with a peculiar deformity of the nose.

HPI

The patient has a history of **nasal stuffiness** and bloody nasal discharge; he also complains of **loss of libido.**

PE

Leonine facies (thickened facial and forehead skin); loss of eyebrows and eyelashes (MADAROSIS); scleral nodules; **depressed nasal bridge** ("SADDLE-NOSE" DEFORMITY); gynecomastia; **testicular atrophy**; numerous **symmetrical, hypopigmented macules with vague edges** and erythematous, smooth, shiny surfaces; skin plaques and nodules; **partial loss of pinprick and temperature sensation** (HYPOESTHESIA); no anhidrotic changes; symmetrically **enlarged ulnar and common peroneal nerves.**

Labs

CBC: mild anemia. ESR elevated; slit skin smears reveal **numerous acid-fast bacilli** on modified ZN staining.

Micro Pathology

Dermis massively and diffusely infiltrated with **foamy histiocytes with bacilli and globi** (masses of acid-fast bacilli) containing Virchow giant cells; bacilli found only rarely in epidermis and in subepidermal "**clear zone**"; epidermis thinned out with flattening of rete ridges.

Treatment

Multidrug therapy with **rifampicin, dapsone, and clofazimine.**

Discussion

The discovery of one or more of the following is pathognomonic of leprosy: (1) **anesthetic skin lesions** (found in all tuberculoid and many lepromatous cases); (2) **thickening of one or more nerves** (found in many lepromatous and some tuberculoid cases); and (3) the presence of **acid-fast bacilli in skin smears** (found in all lepromatous and some tuberculoid cases). *Mycobacterium leprae* has not been cultured in vitro thus far. Frequent complications include hand crippling (secondary to nerve damage) and blindness. It is currently believed that in most instances, the mode of transmission is via person-to-person contact.

ID/CC A 26-year-old male from India presents with a **hypopigmented, anesthetic skin patch** over the left side of his face.

HPI He also complains of an occasional "electric current"-like sensation radiating from his left elbow to his hand.

PE Dry, hypopigmented, anesthetic patch over left cheek; left **ulnar nerve enlarged and palpable**; eye, ear, nose, and throat exam normal; testes normal (vs. signs that are often demonstrable in lepromatous leprosy).

Labs Glucose-6-phosphate dehydrogenase (G6PD) levels within normal range (done to prevent dapsone-associated hemolysis); slit skin smears reveal few **acid-fast bacilli**; skin biopsy from patch diagnostic of tuberculoid leprosy.

Gross Pathology **Single or small number of lesions** with macular or raised edges.

Micro Pathology Skin biopsy reveals many well-formed epithelioid granulomas with very **few** acid-fast bacilli.

Treatment Chemotherapy with rifampin and dapsone.

Discussion Caused by *Mycobacterium leprae*, an acid-fast bacillus. The organism has two unique properties: it is thermolabile, growing best at 27°C to 30°C, and it divides very slowly; generation time is 12 to 14 days. Consequently, leprosy in humans typically evolves very slowly. Tuberculoid leprosy predominantly affects the skin with limited nerve involvement (most commonly ulnar and peroneal); **lepromatous leprosy** has diffuse involvement of the skin, eyes, nerves, and upper airway with disfigurement of the hands and face (**leonine facies**).

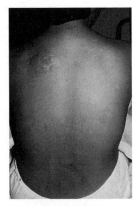

Figure 046A Multiple plaques, nodules and hypopigmented patches.

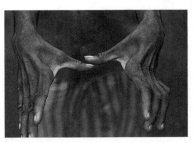

Figure 046B Muscular atrophy and claw hand deformity secondary to bilateral ulnar nerve palsy.

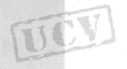

CASE 47

ID/CC   A 35-year-old British **dairy farmer** complains of a high remittent **fever** with chills, severe muscle aches, **decreased urine output**, and **dark-colored urine** for the past 2 days.

HPI   He also complains of an extensive skin rash and nasal bleeding (EPISTAXIS). A careful history reveals that the area in which he works is infested with rodents.

PE   VS: fever; tachycardia; hypotension. PE: **icterus**; extensive hemorrhagic maculopapular skin eruption; **conjunctival suffusion**; lymphadenopathy.

Labs   CBC: leukocytosis with neutrophilia; thrombocytopenia. Mild **hyperbilirubinemia**, predominantly conjugated; **increased alkaline phosphatase; elevated BUN and creatinine.** UA: proteinuria, **casts**, and RBCs. Blood culture (positive during first 10 days of illness) and urine culture (positive after second week of infection) on Fletcher's medium isolated *Leptospira interrogans*; serologic diagnosis (positive during second week of illness): microscopic slide agglutination demonstrated significant titer of antibody to *L. interrogans*.

Imaging   CXR: patchy alveolar infiltrates consistent with alveolar hemorrhage.

Gross Pathology   Severe infection damages both the **liver and kidneys.**

Micro Pathology   Liver biopsy shows focal centrilobular necrosis with focal lymphocytic infiltration and disorganization of liver cell plates together with proliferation of Kupffer cells with cholestasis; kidney biopsy reveals mesangial proliferation with PMN infiltration.

Treatment   IV penicillin; doxycycline for uncomplicated infections; supportive therapy for multiorgan failure.

Discussion   Weil's disease, a severe form of leptospirosis caused by *Leptospira interrogans* complex, is characterized by fever, jaundice, cutaneous and visceral hemorrhages, anemia, azotemia, and altered consciousness; major vectors to humans are rodents. Transmission occurs through direct contact with the blood, tissue, or urine of infected animals. Person-to-person transmission is highly unlikely. Preventive measures include limiting the rodent population and vaccinating animals.

ID/CC   A **neonate died** shortly after birth.

HPI   Review of the medical record reveals history of **refusal to feed**, an extensive **maculopapular skin rash** on his legs and trunk, **respiratory distress**, diarrhea, and seizures shortly after birth.

Discussion   Neonatal listeriosis may occur early or late in neonatal life. Infants may be acutely ill at birth and may die within hours as a result of disseminated listeriosis, which is also called **granulomatosis infantiseptica**. This condition is characterized by **hepatosplenomegaly, thrombocytopenia**, generalized **skin papules**, whitish pharyngeal patches, and **pneumonia**. Commonly, a stained smear of meconium will reveal **gram-positive bacilli**, suggesting the diagnosis.

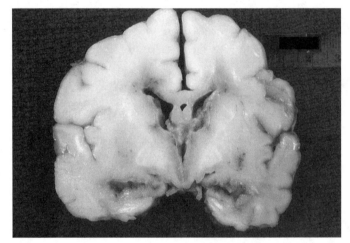

Figure 048 Swollen brain parenchyma with opaque meninges.

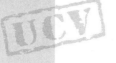

ID/CC   A 2-week-old female is brought to the emergency room because of high fever and convulsions.

HPI   She also has an extensive skin rash on her legs and trunk.

PE   VS: fever. PE: generalized hypotonia; extensive maculopapular skin rash; nuchal rigidity; involuntary flexion of hips when flexing neck (BRUDZINSKI'S SIGN).

Labs   CBC: neutrophilic leukocytosis. LP: elevated CSF cell count (750 cells/mL), mostly neutrophils; elevated CSF protein; low CSF sugar. Gram-positive, facultative, intracellular, nonsporulating motile bacilli on Gram stain and culture.

Gross Pathology   Purulent meningitis.

Micro Pathology   Bacillus provokes both acute suppurative reaction with neutrophilic infiltration and chronic granuloma formation with focal necrosis.

Treatment   IV antibiotics (high-dose ampicillin).

Discussion   Listeriosis is caused by *Listeria monocytogenes*. Bacterial infection may occur early (acquired in utero) or later (drinking contaminated milk) in neonatal life. May be rapidly fatal if disseminated. Also occurs in adults immunocompromised by disease (e.g., renal disease or HIV). *Escherichia coli* and group B streptococcus are two other common causes of neonatal meningitis.

ID/CC   A 12-year-old male presents with **fatigue, fever,** headache, **fleeting joint pain,** and a **reddish rash** on his trunk and left leg of 1 week's duration.

HPI   The patient is a native of **Connecticut** and attended a summer camp in the state's national park 2 weeks ago. He recalls having noticed a **tick bite** on his leg about 2 weeks ago.

PE   VS: fever. PE: red macule on site of bite that has grown circumferentially; **active border and central clearing** (ERYTHEMA CHRONICUM MIGRANS); femoral lymphadenopathy; mild neck stiffness; normal CNS exam.

Labs   **Positive IgM ELISA** for *Borrelia burgdorferi*; diagnosis confirmed by Western blot assay. ECG: normal. LP: lymphocytic pleocytosis; increased proteins. *B. burgdorferi* grown on Noguchi medium.

Gross Pathology   Erythema chronicum migrans (ECM) is characteristic of Lyme disease; must be minimum of 5 cm in diameter for diagnosis to be made; center may desquamate, ulcerate, or necrose; satellite lesions sometimes seen; may spontaneously disappear with time.

Treatment   **Doxycycline**; amoxicillin; ceftriaxone.

Discussion   The most common disease transmitted by vectors in the United States, Lyme disease is caused by *Borrelia burgdorferi*, a spirochete, and is transmitted through *Ixodes* species tick bites. Ticks acquire *B. burgdorferi* from deer mice, which are the natural reservoir. There are three recognized stages: stage 1 consists of ECM and constitutional symptoms; stage 2, cardiac or neurologic involvement; and stage 3, persistent migratory arthritis, synovitis, and **atrophic patches on the distal extremities** (ACRODERMATITIS CHRONICUM ATROPHICANS).

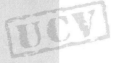
ID/CC
A 25-year-old male complains of swollen, **tender masses in his groin** and very painful **genital ulcers** of 1 week's duration.

HPI
The patient admits to having had **unprotected sex** with multiple partners.

PE
Swollen, erythematous, tender **inguinal nodes**, usually bilateral, with draining sinuses (INGUINAL ADENITIS, BUBOES); multiple small genital lesions.

Labs
Inguinal node biopsy diagnostic; **positive complement fixation test; positive immunofluorescence test.**

Gross Pathology
Primary lesion is ulcerated nodule; gives rise to **inguinal bubo**, an enlarged lymph node sometimes characterized by fistulous tract formation; balanitis, phimosis, and rectal involvement with stricture may also be present.

Micro Pathology
Neutrophilic infiltration of primary lesion with areas of necrosis; lymphoid hyperplasia of lymph nodes with foci of macrophage accumulation; abscess formation with fibrosis.

Treatment
Doxycycline; erythromycin.

Discussion
Lymphogranuloma venereum is an STD that is due to *Chlamydia trachomatis* (**L1, L2, L3**). Counseling should be given about other STDs (e.g., AIDS, syphilis, gonorrhea).

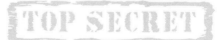

ID/CC   A 50-year-old white male develops **sudden fever with chills**, pain in the back and extremities, and **neck stiffness**; he vomited six times and had a **convulsion** prior to admission.

HPI   The patient is a **heavy smoker** and is **diabetic. Two weeks ago**, he had a URI. He is also very sensitive to light (PHOTOPHOBIA).

PE   Markedly reduced mental status (OBTUNDED); petechial rash over trunk and abdomen; **nuchal and spinal rigidity; positive Kernig's and Brudzinski's signs**; no focal neurologic deficits.

Labs   LP: **elevated pressure; cloudy CSF; elevated protein; markedly decreased glucose; high cell count with mostly WBCs.** CSF Gram stain reveals **gram-positive diplococci.** Spinal fluid culture grows **Streptococcus pneumoniae.**

Imaging   CT/MR, brain: **meningeal thickening** and enhancement.

Gross Pathology   Pia-arachnoid congestion results from inflammatory infiltrate; thin layer of pus forms and promotes adhesions while obstructing normal CSF flow (can cause hydrocephalus); brain covered with purulent exudate, most heavily on base.

Treatment   Early empiric high-dose IV antibiotics; cefotaxime; vancomycin; high-dose steroids.

Discussion   Bacterial meningitis is a pyogenic infection of the CNS that requires prompt treatment. *Streptococcus pneumoniae* is the most common cause of adult meningitis.

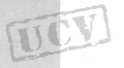

CASE 53

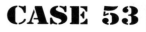

ID/CC

A 4-year-old female presents with a 1-week history of **fever**, severe **headache, irritability**, and **malaise**; 2 days ago she developed **neck stiffness**, and her parents report **projectile vomiting** over the past 24 hours.

HPI

The child is also very sensitive to light (PHOTOPHOBIA). She is fully immunized and has no history of ear, nose, and throat infection, skin rashes, dog bites, or foreign travel.

PE

VS: fever. PE: irritability; resistance to being touched or moved; minimal papilledema of fundus; no focal neurologic signs; no cranial nerve deficits; positive **Kernig's** and **Brudzinski's** signs.

Labs

CBC: **neutrophilic leukocytosis**. LP: increased pressure; **cloudy CSF; neutrophilic pleocytosis; decreased glucose; increased protein; gram-negative coccobacilli**. Negative ZN and India ink staining; normal serum electrolytes; on chocolate agar, blood culture grew *Haemophilus influenzae*; negative Mantoux.

Imaging

CT/MR, brain: **meningeal thickening** and enhancement.

Gross Pathology

Abundant accumulation of purulent exudate between pia mater and arachnoid; meningeal thickening; cloudy to frankly purulent CSF.

Micro Pathology

Intense neutrophilic infiltrate.

Treatment

IV antibiotics (ampicillin, cefotaxime); consider steroids.

Discussion

A pyogenic infection of the nervous system primarily affecting the meninges, bacterial meningitis is most commonly caused by pneumococcus (*Streptococcus pneumoniae*, associated with sickle cell anemia), meningococcus (*Neisseria meningitidis*, associated with a petechial skin rash), and *H. influenzae* (most commonly in children). It is less commonly caused by enterobacteria, *Streptococcus* species, *Staphylococcus* species (due to dental infection), and anaerobic organisms (due to trauma).

ID/CC

A 6-year-old **male** being treated for **primary pulmonary tuberculosis** presents with **diplopia**, increasing drowsiness, irritability, and unexplained, recurrent **vomiting**.

HPI

The child has had a low-grade fever, loss of appetite, and a persistent headache over the past few weeks.

PE

VS: fever. PE: stuporous; signs of meningeal irritation noted (**neck rigidity, Kernig's sign**); **CN III and IV palsy** on right side; funduscopy reveals **papilledema**.

Labs

LP (guarded): CSF under **increased pressure** and **turbid**; on standing, a "cobweb" coagulum formed at center of tube; CSF studies reveal **lymphocytic pleocytosis**, greatly **elevated protein**, and **low sugar**; ZN staining of CSF coagulum reveals presence of **acid-fast bacilli**; radiometric culture yields *Mycobacterium tuberculosis*.

Imaging

CT: suggests **basal exudates**, **inflammatory granulomas**, and a **communicating hydrocephalus**; striking meningeal enhancement noted in postcontrast studies.

Gross Pathology

Meningeal surface covered with yellowish-gray exudates and tubercles that are most numerous at base of brain and along the course of the middle cerebral artery; subarachnoid space and arachnoid villi obliterated (leading to poor absorption of CSF and hence a communicating hydrocephalus).

Micro Pathology

Subarachnoid space contains gelatinous exudate of chronic inflammatory cells, obliterating cisterns, and encasing cranial nerves; well-formed **granulomas** occasionally seen, most often at base of brain; arteries running through subarachnoid space show "obliterative endarteritis."

Treatment

Antituberculous therapy with rifampin, isoniazid, ethambutol and pyrazinamide; steroids; ventriculoperitoneal shunt to relieve hydrocephalus.

Discussion

Tuberculous infection reaches the meninges through the hematogenous route, resulting in a clinically subacute form of meningitis; it is often complicated by cranial nerve palsies, a communicating hydrocephalus, decerebrate posturing, convulsions, coma, and death.

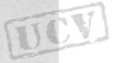

CASE 55

ID/CC A 12-year-old white female is brought to the emergency room because of sudden **fever** with **chills, severe headache,** pain in the extremities and back, **stiff neck,** and generalized rash; she also **fainted** while in school.

HPI She had been well until admission, with no relevant history. In the emergency room, she **vomits bright red blood** twice.

PE VS: tachycardia; hypotension (BP 70/50). PE: altered sensorium; pallor; moist, cold skin; nuchal rigidity and positive Kernig's sign; **petechial rash** all over body; minimal papilledema on funduscopic exam; no focal neurologic signs.

Labs Hypoglycemia. Lytes: **hyponatremia; hyperkalemia.** CBC/PBS: thrombocytopenia; **neutrophilic leukocytosis.** LP: **CSF** cloudy and under increased pressure; increased proteins; low sugar. **Gram-negative diplococci** (*Neisseria meningitidis*) **seen within and outside WBCs** on Gram stain; negative India ink and ZN stain; growth of meningococci later revealed on blood culture.

Imaging CT, head: normal. CT, abdomen: bilateral adrenal hemorrhage.

Gross Pathology **Bilateral adrenal hemorrhagic necrosis;** skin necrosis; pyogenic meningitis.

Micro Pathology Meningeal hyperemia with abundant purulent exudate; diplococcus-containing PMNs; acute hemorrhagic necrosis of adrenal glands.

Treatment Steroid replacement; IV fluids; dopamine; IV penicillin or ceftriaxone; prophylactic rifampin or ciprofloxacin for close contacts.

Discussion Meningococcemia is a **fulminant disease** caused by several groups of *Neisseria meningitidis*; the cause of death is adrenal necrosis with vascular collapse. A meningococcal vaccine is available. Also known as **Waterhouse–Friderichsen syndrome.**

ID/CC A 20-year-old male college student presents with a **productive cough**, headache, **malaise**, runny nose, and **fever**.

HPI He has a history of sore throat preceding the onset of the **cough, which initially was nonproductive**.

PE VS: fever. PE: mild respiratory distress; auscultation reveals fine to medium rales over right lower lobe.

Labs Gram stain of sputum negative; routine cultures of both blood and sputum negative. CBC: **leukocyte count normal**. Fourfold rise in complement fixation titer in paired sera; **cold agglutinin titer > 1:128**.

Imaging CXR: patchy alveolar infiltrates involving right lower lobe; appears worse than the clinical picture.

Gross Pathology Unilateral lower lobe pneumonia with firm, red pulmonary parenchyma in affected areas.

Micro Pathology Bronchial mucosa congested and edematous; inflammatory response consists of perivascular lymphocytes initially and PMNs later in infection. **Organism lacks cell wall** (thus penicillins and cephalosporins are ineffective).

Treatment Erythromycin.

Discussion *Mycoplasma pneumoniae* is the **most common cause of primary atypical pneumonia**. Transmission is by droplet spread; rapidly infects those living in close quarters.

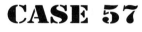

CASE 57

BACTERIOLOGY

ID/CC	A 14-year-old **malnourished child** died soon after hospitalization due to an **extensive small bowel rupture and shock**.

HPI	He had presented to the emergency room with **massive bloody diarrhea**. His history at admission revealed the presence of abdominal pain, fever, and diarrhea of a few days' duration; his symptoms had developed **after he ate leftover meat** at a fast-food restaurant.

PE	He was dehydrated, pale, and hypotensive at time of admission and developed signs of peritonitis and shock shortly before his death.

Labs	Culture and exam of necrotizing intestinal lesions isolated *Clostridium perfringens* type C producing beta toxin.

Gross Pathology	Autopsy revealed ruptured small intestine, mucosal ulcerations, and **gas production** in the wall.

Micro Pathology	Microscopic exam revealed necrosis and acute inflammation in the ileum.

Treatment	Patient died despite aggressive fluid and electrolyte replacement, bowel decompression, and antibiotic therapy (penicillin, clindamycin, or doxycycline); surgery had been planned in view of rupture of the small bowel.

Discussion	Necrotizing enterocolitis is a condition affecting poorly nourished persons who suddenly feast on meat (pigbel). It is associated with *Clostridium perfringens* type C and **beta enterotoxin**; beta toxin paralyzes the villi and causes friability and necrosis of the bowel wall. Immunization of children in New Guinea with beta-toxoid vaccine has dramatically decreased the incidence of the disease.

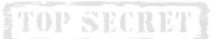

ID/CC   A 50-year-old diabetic male presents with **fever, pain, and a necrotizing swelling** over his left leg.

HPI   His symptoms began about a week ago with redness and swelling of the left leg followed by bronze discoloration of the skin and the appearance of hemorrhagic bullae.

PE   Extensive cutaneous **gangrene** observed over left leg with many ruptured bullae; black necrotic eschar with surrounding erythema resembles a third-degree burn.

Labs   Swab staining reveals presence of chains of gram-positive cocci; culture isolated **β-hemolytic group A streptococcus** (*Streptococcus pyogenes*).

Micro Pathology   Biopsy specimen reveals areas of necrosis in dermis and subcutaneous fat, infiltration with PMNs, and vasculitis and thrombosis in vessels in the superficial fascia.

Treatment   Treatment includes rapid **surgical excision of necrotic tissue** in combination with appropriate **antibiotics**; **penicillin G** is drug of choice for streptococcal infection.

Discussion   Streptococcal gangrene is a group A streptococcal cellulitis that rapidly progresses to gangrene of the subcutaneous tissue and necrosis of the overlying skin; the disease process usually involves an extremity. Necrotizing fasciitis is also recognized as a polymicrobial infection that is caused by aerobes and anaerobes ("SYNERGISTIC NECROTIZING CELLULITIS"). Infection spreads quickly through various fascial planes, the venous system, and lymphatics. Predisposing etiologies include surgery, trauma, and diabetes.

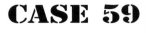

ID/CC　　A 7-year-old male who has been hospitalized for treatment of **acute lymphocytic leukemia** complains of **copious watery diarrhea**, right lower quadrant **abdominal pain**, and **fever**.

HPI　　He was diagnosed as **neutropenic** (due to aggressive cytotoxic chemotherapy) a few days ago.

PE　　VS: fever; tachycardia; tachypnea. PE: pallor; sternal tenderness; axillary lymphadenopathy; hepatosplenomegaly; abdominal distention; moderate dehydration.

Labs　　CBC: severe **neutropenia**; anemia; thrombocytopenia. PBS and bone marrow studies suggest he is in remission; blood culture grows *Clostridium septicum*.

Imaging　　CT, abdomen: **thickening of cecal wall**.

Gross Pathology　　Mucosal ulcers and inflammation in **ileocecal region** of small intestine.

Treatment　　Aggressive **supportive measures**; surgical intervention; appropriate **antibiotics** (penicillin G, ampicillin, or clindamycin).

Discussion　　Neutropenic enterocolitis is a fulminant form of necrotizing enteritis that occurs in neutropenic patients; neutropenia is often related to cyclic neutropenia, leukemia, aplastic anemia, or chemotherapy. In postmortem exams of patients who have died of leukemia, infections of the cecal area (TYPHLITIS) are frequently found; *Clostridium septicum* is the most common organism isolated from the blood of such patients.

TOP SECRET

CASE 60

ID/CC A 45-year-old white male undergoing **chemotherapy** for Hodgkin's lymphoma is brought to the emergency room by his wife because of shortness of breath and cyanosis.

HPI For the past **3 months**, he has been complaining of intermittent weakness, fever with chills, and foul-smelling, thick **greenish sputum**.

PE VS: fever (38°C); tachypnea; tachycardia. PE: pallor; mild cyanosis; localized dullness with bronchial breathing; diminished breath sounds over left lower lobe.

Labs CBC: leukocytosis with neutrophilia; anemia. Sputum culture reveals **gram-positive, filamentous, partially acid-fast** staining bacteria (due to *Nocardia*).

Imaging CXR: nodular infiltrate in left lower lobe with air-fluid level (abscess) and left pleural effusion.

Gross Pathology Lung lesions or disseminated lesions (brain, liver, kidney, subcutaneous tissue) consist of necrotic centers within regions of consolidation and abscess formation resembling pyogenic pneumonia.

Micro Pathology Consolidation of alveoli with pus formation (exudate of PMNs and fibrin) and surrounding granulomatous reaction.

Treatment Six-month course of TMP-SMX; surgery.

Discussion A chronic bacterial infection seen in diabetics, leukemia and lymphoma patients, and **immunocompromised patients**, nocardiosis usually involves the lungs with possible dissemination to the brain, subcutaneous tissue, and other organs. It is caused by *Nocardia asteroides*, a branching, aerobic, gram-positive organism that is weakly acid fast and is sometimes confused with *Mycobacterium tuberculosis*.

TOP SECRET

CASE 61

ID/CC A 60-year-old male who was hospitalized following a stroke presents with a high-grade **fever with chills** and obtundation.

HPI He had been **catheterized due to urinary incontinence and was receiving cephalosporin** for treatment of aspiration pneumonitis.

PE VS: fever.

Labs Blood culture grew *Enterococcus fecalis* (morphologically indistinguishable from streptococci and immunologically similar to members of group D streptococci, the enterococci are metabolically unique in their ability to resist heat, bile, and 6.5% NaCl); urine culture also isolated *Streptococcus fecalis*.

Treatment **Ampicillin with gentamicin** (**vancomycin** can be substituted for ampicillin in patients with penicillin allergies).

Discussion Enterococci constitute a relatively common cause of UTIs, wound infections, and peritonitis and intra-abdominal abscesses; they have also become an increasingly prominent cause of **bacteremia**, which usually originates from a **focus in the urinary tract or abdomen**. The incidence of nosocomial bacteremias caused by these organisms is also increasing, particularly in patients who have received cephalosporins or other broad-spectrum antibiotics. All clinically significant isolates should be subjected to testing for β-lactamase production, high-level **aminoglycoside resistance**, and **vancomycin resistance** to determine if an alternative therapy is necessary. Infections caused by enterococci that produce β-lactamase are treated with an antimicrobial agent that combines a penicillin with a β-lactamase inhibitor; infections caused by strains that are highly resistant to aminoglycosides are treated with vancomycin.

BACTERIOLOGY

ID/CC
A 4-year-old white male presents with fever, chills, malaise, **pain**, and **immobility of the right knee** of 1 week's duration.

HPI
Two weeks ago the child fell while playing, but no abnormality was found by the school nurse.

PE
Overlying skin **warm and red**; **swelling** of distal third of thigh and knee; **tenderness** on palpation.

Labs
CBC: leukocytosis. **Elevated ESR**. Gram stain and culture confirm diagnosis and isolate pathogen.

Imaging
XR, plain: early findings include soft tissue edema and thin line running parallel to diaphysis **(periosteal thickening)**; later findings include bone erosion, subperiosteal abscess with periostitis, and sequestrum formation (due to detached necrotic cortical bone); involucrum formation (laminated periosteal reaction). MR: marrow edema; abscess. Indium-labeled WBC, scan: hot spot.

Gross Pathology
New osteoblastic periosteal bone formation (INVOLUCRUM); **trapping of detached necrotic bone by involucrum** (SEQUESTRUM); isolated localized abscess (BRODIE'S ABSCESS); sinus tract formation, draining pus to skin.

Micro Pathology
Purulent exudate formation, usually metaphyseal, with ischemic necrosis of bone due to increased pressure of pus in rigid bone walls; vascular thrombosis.

Treatment
IV antibiotics according to sensitivity; **surgical debridement**.

Discussion
Osteomyelitis is an acute pyogenic bone infection which, if left untreated, produces functional incapacity and deformities. The most common pathogen is ***Staphylococcus aureus***; less frequently *Streptococcus* and enterobacteria are involved. In sickle cell anemia *Escherichia coli* and *Salmonella* species are seen; diabetics are at risk for *Pseudomonas* infection. Immunocompromised patients may show *Sporothrix schenckii* osteomyelitis; human bites, anaerobes; puncture wounds, *Pseudomonas aeruginosa*; and cat-bite wounds, *Pasteurella multocida*.

ID/CC   A 20-year-old male swimmer complains of severe **pain** and **itching** in the right ear that is associated with a slight amount of **yellowish** (PURULENT) **discharge**.

HPI   The patient has no previous history of discharge from the ear and no history of associated deafness or tinnitus.

PE   Red, swollen area seen in right external auditory meatus that is partially obliterating the lumen; **movement of tragus** is exquisitely **painful** (TRAGAL SIGN).

Labs   Gram stain of aural swab reveals presence of gram-negative rods; culture isolates *Pseudomonas aeruginosa*.

Gross Pathology   Red, swollen area seen in cartilaginous part of external auditory meatus; when visualized, tympanic membrane is erythematous and moves normally with pneumatic otoscopy (vs. acute otitis media).

Treatment   **Eardrops** (either a combination of polymyxin, neomycin, and hydrocortisone or ofloxacin); gentle removal of debris in ear.

Discussion   Otitis externa is most common in summer months and is thought to arise from a change in the milieu of the external auditory meatus by increased alkalization and excessive moisture; this leads to bacterial overgrowth, most commonly with gram-negative rods such as *Pseudomonas* (also causes malignant otitis externa) and *Proteus* or fungi such as *Aspergillus*.

ID/CC An 18-month-old white female presents with **irritability** together with a bilateral, profuse, and foul-smelling **ear discharge** of 2 months' duration.

HPI The patient had **recurrent URIs** last year, but her mother did not administer the complete course of antibiotics. The patient's mother has a history of feeding her child while lying down.

PE Bilateral greenish-white ear discharge; **perforated tympanic membranes** in anteroinferior quadrant of both ears; **diminished mobility of tympanic membrane** on pneumatic otoscopy.

Labs Gram-negative coccobacilli on Gram stain of discharge from tympanocentesis; *Haemophilus influenzae* seen on culture.

Gross Pathology Possible complications include **ingrowth of squamous epithelium on upper middle ear** (CHOLESTEATOMA) if long-standing; conductive hearing loss; mastoiditis; and brain abscess.

Micro Pathology Hyperemia and edema of inner ear and throat mucosa; hyperemia of tympanic membrane; deposition of cholesterol crystals in keratinized epidermoid cells in cholesteatoma.

Treatment Keep ear dry; **amoxicillin-clavulanic acid**; surgical drainage for severe otalgia; myringoplasty.

Discussion Otitis media is the most common pediatric bacterial infection and is caused by *Escherichia coli, Staphylococcus aureus,* and *Klebsiella pneumoniae* in neonates; in older children it is usually caused by pneumococcus (*Streptococcus pneumoniae*), *H. influenzae, Moraxella catarrhalis,* and group A streptococcus. Resistant strains are becoming increasingly common.

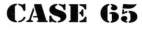

CASE 65

ID/CC   A 9-year-old male is admitted for an evaluation of a **suspected** underlying **immune deficiency**.

HPI   He has been hospitalized and treated several times for **recurrent** life-threatening **septicemia due to** *Streptococcus pneumoniae,* **meningococcus**, and *Haemophilus influenzae*. Careful history reveals that a few years ago he underwent an emergency **splenectomy** following traumatic splenic rupture in a motor vehicle accident.

PE   Left paramedian postsurgical scar seen on abdomen.

Labs   Reduced IgM levels; **reduced antibody production when challenged with particulate antigens**; PBS reveals **Howell–Jolly bodies**.

Imaging   US, abdomen: **spleen is absent**.

Treatment   **Pneumococcal vaccine and prophylactic antibiotics** (penicillin, amoxicillin, TMP-SMX).

Discussion   Patients who have undergone **splenectomy or** who are **functionally asplenic** are at increased **risk for overwhelming bacteremia**; pathogens include **organisms that possess a polysaccharide capsule**, such as meningococcus, *Staphylococcus*, the DF2 bacillus, and, especially, *Streptococcus pneumoniae* and *Haemophilus influenzae* type B. Such **functionally asplenic** patients include individuals with **sickle cell disease** and those who have undergone **splenic irradiation**. **Pneumococcal vaccine** is indicated in all patients who have undergone splenectomy, particularly children and adolescents.

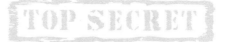

ID/CC   A 12-year-old girl arrives in the emergency room with **pain, swelling, and limited motion** of her left hand; she also complains of fever and chills.

HPI   The girl was **bitten by a cat** yesterday while playing at a friend's house.

PE   Hand is erythematous, **shiny**, and **markedly edematous**; on palpation, hand is **tender** with fluctuation (cellulitis); limited passive and active motion; yellowish-green **purulent fluid** drains from wound; left epitrochlear and axillary **lymphadenitis** without lymphangitis.

Labs   **Gram-negative rods with bipolar staining** of abscess aspirate; **catalase and oxidase positive** (*Pasteurella multocida*).

Imaging   Local wound care; **tetanus** and **rabies prophylaxis**; **polymicrobial antibiotic coverage** with amoxicillin/clavulanate or tetracyclines; meticulous follow-up evaluation for complications.

Treatment   **Incision and drainage, amoxicillin/clavulanate**; tetracycline; penicillin.

Discussion   *Pasteurella multocida* is the most common bacterium isolated from cat bite wounds and may progress to **osteomyelitis**. Human bite infections are most commonly caused by *Eikenella corrodens* and are treated with penicillin.

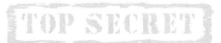

ID/CC
A 28-year-old **sexually active woman** presents with crampy **lower abdominal pain**, yellowish **vaginal discharge**, and general malaise.

HPI
She also complains of continuous low-grade fever and reveals that the **pain** is **exacerbated during and immediately after menstruation** (CONGESTIVE DYSMENORRHEA). She uses a copper **intrauterine device** for contraception.

PE
VS: low-grade fever. PE: **lower abdominal tenderness**; bimanual pelvic exam demonstrates **purulent vaginal discharge**, bilateral **adnexal tenderness**, and pain on movement of cervix (MUCOPURULENT CERVICITIS).

Labs
CBC: leukocytosis with left shift. Increased ESR; endocervical swab sent for microscopic exam; staining and culture revealed combined infection with *Neisseria gonorrhoeae* (cultured on Thayer-Martin medium) and *Chlamydia trachomatis* (identified on cell culture, immunofluorescence, and antigen capture assay); **laparoscopy** ("gold standard" for diagnosis) confirmed diagnosis.

Imaging
USG: free pelvic fluid, dilated tubular structure in adnexa.

Gross Pathology
Erythema and swelling of fallopian tubes on laparoscopy; seropurulent exudate noted on surface of tubes from fimbriated end.

Micro Pathology
Endocervical swab reveals increased neutrophils and gram-negative diplococci seen both intra- and extracellularly; cervical biopsy reveals inclusions containing *Chlamydia* within columnar cells.

Treatment
Antibiotic therapy with cefoxitin (for *N. gonorrhoeae*) and doxycycline (for chlamydial infection); male partners must be treated for STDs.

Discussion
Pelvic inflammatory disease usually occurs as a primary infection that ascends from the lower genital tract due to STDs caused by *Neisseria gonorrhoeae* and *Chlamydia trachomatis*. Sequelae of PID include peritonitis; intestinal obstruction due to adhesions; dissemination leading to arthritis, meningitis, and endocarditis; chronic pelvic pain; infertility; ectopic pregnancy; and recurrent PID.

ID/CC   A 20-year-old Asian woman presents with complaints of infertility and heavy bleeding during menses (MENORRHAGIA).

HPI   She was treated for pulmonary tuberculosis a few years ago. She has been unable to conceive despite unprotected intercourse for the past 2 years. Her husband's semen analysis is normal.

PE   On pelvic exam, small, fixed adnexal masses are palpable that are matted and fixed to uterus ("FROZEN PELVIS").

Labs   Culture of endometrial curettings yields *Mycobacterium tuberculosis*; histologic examination of curettings reveals presence of characteristic tubercles; Mantoux skin test strongly positive.

Imaging   CXR: left apical fibrosis (evidence of old healed pulmonary tuberculosis). (Hysterosalpingography [HSG] is contraindicated in a proven case of tuberculosis. When done in asymptomatic cases, HSG yields certain typical findings, including a rigid, nonperistaltic, pipelike tube; beading and variation in filling density; calcification of the tube; cornual block; jagged fluffiness of the tubal outline; and vascular or lymphatic extravasation of the dye.)

Gross Pathology   Tubes are enlarged, thickened, and tortuous; examination of uterus reveals evidence of synechiae and adhesions (leading to Asherman's syndrome).

Micro Pathology   Microscopic exam of tubes, ovaries, and endometrium reveals evidence of granulomas with giant cells and caseation.

Treatment   Four-drug therapy with isoniazid, pyrazinamide, ethambutol, and rifampicin; pyridoxine to prevent isoniazid-induced deficiency.

Discussion   Genital tuberculosis is almost always secondary to a focus elsewhere in the body, with the bloodstream by far the most common method of spread. The fallopian tubes are the most frequently involved part of the genital tract, followed by the uterus. Ninety percent of patients are cured with chemotherapy, although only 10% regain fertility.

ID/CC   A 25-year-old male complains of **midepigastric pain** that usually begins **1 to 2 hours after eating** and occasionally awakens him at night.

HPI   The patient has been diagnosed with **duodenal ulcers** several times in the past, but his **symptoms have** consistently **recurred** even after therapy with H$_2$ blockers, antacids, and sucralfate.

PE   VS: stable. PE: pallor; epigastric tenderness on deep palpation.

Labs   CBC: normocytic, normochromic anemia. Stool positive for occult blood; *Helicobacter pylori* antibody detected in serum; *H. pylori* antigen detected in stool.

Imaging   UGI: ulcerations in antrum of stomach and duodenum; antral biopsy specimens yield **positive urease test**.

Gross Pathology   Grossly round ulcer (may also be oval) seen as sharply punched-out defect with relatively straight walls and slight overhanging of mucosal margin (heaped-up margin is characteristic of a malignant lesion); smooth and clean ulcer base.

Micro Pathology   No evidence of malignancy; **antral biopsies** reveal presence of **chronic mucosal inflammation**; *H. pylori* identified on Giemsa stain.

Treatment   *Helicobacter pylori* eradication employing one proton pump inhibitor (e.g., omeprazole) and two antibiotics (e.g., amoxicillin and clarithromycin).

Discussion   *Helicobacter pylori* grows overlying the antral gastric mucosal cells; 40% of healthy individuals and approximately 50% of patients with peptic disease harbor this organism. Although *H. pylori* **does not breach the epithelial barrier**, colonization of the antral mucosal layer by this organism is associated with structural alterations of the gastric mucosa and hence with a high prevalence of antral gastritis. Despite the fact that *H. pylori* does not grow on duodenal mucosa, it is strongly associated with duodenal ulcer, and eradication of the organism in patients with refractory peptic ulcer disease decreases the risk of recurrence.

ID/CC   A 9-year-old male complains of **pain during swallowing** (ODYNOPHAGIA) for 2 days, accompanied by muscle aches, headache, and fever.

HPI   He has otherwise been in good health and has no history of cough, runny nose, or itchy eyes.

PE   VS: fever. PE: moderate erythema of pharynx; enlarged, **erythematous tonsils** covered with white **exudate**; tender cervical adenopathy.

Labs   CBC: neutrophilic leukocytosis. Rapid streptococcal antigen test positive; *Streptococcus pyogenes* isolated on throat swab and culture.

Gross Pathology   Hyperemia and swelling of upper respiratory tract mucosa; cryptic enlargement of tonsils with purulent exudate; enlargement of regional lymph nodes.

Micro Pathology   Acute inflammatory response with polymorphonuclear infiltrate, hyperemia and edema with pus formation; hyperplasia of regional lymph nodes; dilatation of sinusoids.

Treatment   Oral penicillin V.

Discussion   Streptococcal pharyngitis is an acute bacterial infection produced by gram-positive **cocci in chains** (*Streptococcus*); pharyngitis is most commonly caused by group A streptococcus. Complications due to immune-mediated cross-reactivity and molecular mimicking may include glomerulonephritis and rheumatic fever.

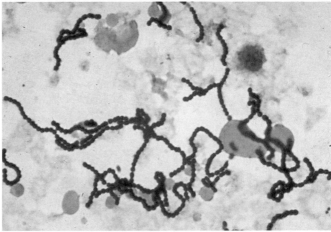

Figure 070 Long chains of gram-positive cocci.

ID/CC

A 44-year-old male archaeologist presents with **high fever, malaise,** intense **headache, severe myalgia,** and **painful swelling in the inguinal region.**

HPI

He recently returned from a trip to **Arizona.**

PE

VS: tachycardia; fever. PE: drowsy looking; no meningeal signs; pustule seen at site of an **insect bite** on left upper arm; **inguinal lymph nodes enlarged, fluctuant, and tender** (BUBOES); no lesion on external genitalia.

Labs

CBC/PBS: normal; no malarial parasites. Gram-negative bacilli with "**safety pin**" appearance seen in aspirates from buboes; culture of aspirate reveals *Yersinia pestis.*

Gross Pathology

Enlarged lymph nodes are necrotic and suppurative; pneumonic form shows lobar consolidation.

Micro Pathology

Numerous organisms in suppurative and necrotic lymph tissue.

Treatment

Hospitalization with standard precautions; antibiotic therapy with **streptomycine.**

Discussion

Plague is usually acquired after contact with **rodents and fleas** in endemic areas (southwestern United States). Septic shock, pneumonia, DIC, and vascular collapse are life-threatening sequelae. The **pneumonic form** of the disease has a high fatality rate and requires the institution of **droplet precautions** for hospitalized patients along with prompt administration of **doxycycline prophylaxis** to their contacts.

ID/CC An 11-year-old white male presents with a high-grade fever, a productive, **blood-tinged** cough, **mucoid sputum**, and **pleuritic left-sided chest pain** of a few days' duration.

HPI The child had previously been well and is fully immunized.

PE VS: fever; tachypnea. PE: use of accessory respiratory muscles; central trachea; decreased left respiratory excursion; **increased vocal fremitus in left infrascapular area with dullness to percussion; bronchial breathing** with coarse crackles heard over left lung area.

Labs CBC: increased WBC count; preponderance of neutrophils. ABGs: hypoxemia without hypercapnia. **Gram-positive diplococci in sputum**; α-hemolytic colonies of gram-positive diplococci (*Streptococcus pneumoniae*) on blood agar culture.

Imaging CXR: **homogenous opacification of left lower lobe** (LOBAR CONSOLIDATION) with small left pleural effusion.

Gross Pathology Consolidation of lung parenchyma passes through four stages: congestion and edema, red hepatization, gray hepatization, and resolution.

Micro Pathology Vascular dilatation with hyperemia and alveolar edema; PMNs rich in purulent exudate; fibrin deposition; hardening of lung parenchyma with fibrin clotting inside alveoli (consolidation).

Treatment Parenteral antibiotic therapy; empiric initial choice of ceftriaxone and/or azithromycin followed by culture sensitivity–guided treatment; supportive respiratory therapy; monitoring with clinical and radiologic response.

Discussion *Streptococcus pneumoniae* is the most common cause of community-acquired pneumonia and produces typical lobar pneumonia. Predisposing conditions include prior splenectomy or nonfunctional spleen, HIV infection, sickle cell anemia, and alcoholism.

TOP SECRET

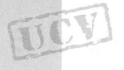

ID/CC   A 32-year-old **HIV-positive male** presents with **progressively increasing dyspnea** over the past 3 weeks.

HPI   He also complains of a **dry**, painful **cough**, marked **fatigue**, and a continuous **low-grade fever**. He has been noncompliant with cotrimoxazole prophylaxis.

PE   VS: fever; marked **tachypnea**. PE: pallor; generalized lymphadenopathy; respiratory distress; **intercostal retraction**; mild central cyanosis; nasal flaring; coarse, crepitant rales auscultated at both lung bases.

Labs   ABGs: **hypoxemia out of proportion to clinical findings**. *Pneumocystis carinii* on **methenamine silver stain** of induced sputum or bronchoalveolar lavage; ELISA/Western blot positive for HIV. CBC: **leukopenia** with depressed CD4+ cell count. **Serum LDH typically elevated**.

Imaging   CXR: diffuse, bilaterally symmetrical **interstitial and alveolar infiltration** pattern, predominantly perihilar; no lymphadenopathy or effusion.

Gross Pathology   Congestion and consolidation of lungs with hypoaeration.

Micro Pathology   Eosinophilic exudate in alveoli with multiple 4- to 6-mm cysts containing oval bodies (MEROZOITES) on lung biopsy or bronchial lavage; *Pneumocystis* abundant on Gomori methenamine silver stain.

Treatment   IV TMP-SMX; alternative antimicrobials for patients sensitive to TMP-SMX include pentamidine, atovaquone, and clindamycin; steroids for severe disease.

Discussion   *Pneumocystis carinii* pneumonia is an opportunistic infection that causes interstitial pneumonia in many **immunocompromised** patients. Traditionally it has been classified as a protozoan; however, *P. carinii* ribosomal RNA indicates that the organism is **fungal**. It is seen in the upper lobes in patients receiving inhaled pentamidine prophylaxis. Treat HIV patients prophylactically with TMP-SMX for *P. carinii* pneumonia if the CD4 count is < 200.

TOP SECRET

ID/CC   A 10-year-old child presents with complaints of acute-onset voiding of tea-colored urine and reduced urinary output.

HPI   The child was treated 1 week ago for streptococcal pyoderma that was confirmed by culture. He also complains of puffiness around the eyes and mild swelling of both feet.

PE   VS: hypertension (BP 140/96); fever; tachycardia. PE: periorbital swelling; mild pitting pedal edema; no ascites or kidney mass palpable.

Labs   CBC: mild leukocytosis. Elevated BUN and creatinine; elevated ASO titer; serum cryoglobulins present. UA: RBC casts; proteinuria. C3 levels reduced in blood.

Gross Pathology   Smooth, reddish-brown cortical surface with numerous petechial hemorrhages.

Micro Pathology   Biopsy shows diffuse glomerulonephritis resulting from proliferation of endothelial, mesangial, and epithelial cells; granular, "starry-sky" pattern of IgG, IgM, and C3 on immunofluorescence; electron microscopy shows subepithelial "humplike" deposits (antigen-antibody complexes).

Treatment   Penicillin if still infected with *Streptococcus*; diuretics, salt and water restriction and antihypertensives.

Discussion   Poststreptococcal glomerulonephritis is a classic immune complex-mediated entity that is associated with acute nephritic syndrome, which develops following infection with nephritogenic group A β-hemolytic streptococci (e.g., types 1, 4, and 12, which are associated with pharyngitis, and types 49, 55, and 57, which are associated with impetigo).

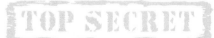

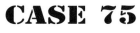

ID/CC

A 25-year-old HIV-negative **homosexual male** presents with rectal burning, itching in the anal region, **diarrhea, tenesmus,** and a **bloody, mucopurulent discharge** per rectum.

HPI

One month ago he was hospitalized with severe **febrile proctocolitis** that was diagnosed as **lymphogranuloma venereum.** He has also been treated several times in the past for amebiasis and shigella colitis and admits to having **receptive anal intercourse.** Further history reveals that his most recent **sexual partner** has been suffering from **urethral pain and discharge.**

PE

Condylomata acuminata noted in perianal distribution; remainder of physical exam normal.

Labs

Gram stain and culture of **rectal swab** reveals gram-negative diplococci identified as *Neisseria gonorrhoeae* on Thayer-Martin medium; urethral swab from partner also isolates *N. gonorrhoeae.*

Imaging

Sigmoidoscopy: proctitis with bloody mucopurulent discharge noted.

Treatment

Ceftriaxone and **doxycycline** (to treat likely concomitant chlamydial infection) for both patient and partner. Most apparent failures of correct antibiotic therapy are in fact due to reinfection; in resistant cases, **spectinomycin, fluoroquinolones,** or other **cephalosporins** can be used.

Discussion

The term **"gay bowel syndrome"** is used in reference to enteric and perirectal infections that are commonly encountered in immune-competent homosexual men; in homosexuals with HIV, opportunistic organisms play a more important role. Common etiologic agents include *Chlamydia trachomatis,* lymphogranuloma venereum serovars, *Neisseria gonorrhoeae,* HSV, *Treponema pallidum,* human papillomavirus, *Campylobacter* species, *Shigella, Entamoeba histolytica,* and *Giardia.*

CASE 76

ID/CC A **25-year-old male** presents with complaints of sudden-onset **fever** and chills, urgency and burning on micturition (DYSURIA), and perineal pain.

HPI His symptoms developed a day after he underwent **urethral dilatation** for a stricture.

PE VS: fever. PE: suprapubic tenderness; rectal exam reveals asymmetrically **swollen**, firm, markedly **tender, hot prostate**; prostatic massage is avoided owing to risk of inducing bacteremia; epididymitis and extreme pain.

Labs Examination and culture of urine and prostatic secretions reveal infection with *Escherichia coli*.

Gross Pathology Edematous gland enlargement with suppuration of entire gland, possibly abscesses and focal areas of necrosis that have coalesced.

Micro Pathology Initially minimal leukocytic infiltration of stroma. Later, necrosis of the gland may lead to gland fibrosis.

Treatment Antibiotic therapy as directed by urine and blood culture sensitivity tests. Abscesses may require surgical drainage.

Discussion *Escherichia coli* **is the most common cause** of acute prostatitis; many cases **follow** the use of **instrumentation for the urethra** and prostate (e.g., catheterization, cystoscopy, urethral dilatation, transurethral resection). Remaining infections are caused by *Klebsiella, Proteus, Pseudomonas*, and *Serratia*. Among the gram positives, enterococcus and *Staphylococcus aureus* are frequent causative organisms.

ID/CC   A **65-year-old male** complains of **recurrent burning,** urgency, and fre-quency of micturition together with vague lower abdominal, lumbar, and perineal pain.

HPI   He also complains of a mucoid urethral discharge. He was previously diagnosed via ultrasound with **benign prostatic hypertrophy** but does not report any severe symptoms of prostatism; his medical history reveals **frequent UTIs** due to *Escherichia coli.*

PE   VS: stable; no fever. PE: rectal exam reveals **enlarged, nodular prostate;** biopsy obtained to rule out carcinoma.

Labs   Examination and culture of expressed prostatic secretions reveal leuko-cytosis and *E. coli.*

Imaging   IVP/voiding cystourethrogram (to rule out underlying anatomic cause): normal.

Gross Pathology   Enlarged prostate with nodularity and calculi.

Micro Pathology   Chronic inflammation and few PMNs around glands and ducts on biopsy; dilated ducts containing inspissated secretions (CORPORA AMYLACEA).

Treatment   **Antibiotics** (TMP-SMX, carbenicillin, quinolones). High fluid intake and abstinence from alcohol. Recurrences are common.

Discussion   Bacterial prostatitis is usually caused by the same gram-negative bacilli that cause UTIs in females; 80% or more of such infections are caused by *Escherichia coli.* Chronic bacterial prostatitis is **common in elderly males** with prostatic hyperplasia and is a frequent cause of recurrent UTIs in males (most antibiotics poorly penetrate the prostate; hence the bacteria are not totally eradicated and continuously seed the urinary tract).

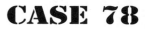

ID/CC　　A 64-year-old male presents with rapidly **progressive dyspnea and fever**.

HPI　　He has a history of orthopnea and paroxysmal nocturnal dyspnea and also reports pink, frothy sputum (HEMOPTYSIS). One month ago he underwent a **bioprosthetic valve replacement** for calcific aortic stenosis. He is not hypertensive and has never had overt cardiac failure in the past.

PE　　VS: fever; hypotension. PE: bilateral basal inspiratory crackles heard; cardiac auscultation suggestive of **aortic incompetence** (early diastolic murmur heard radiating down left sternal edge).

Labs　　CBC: normochromic, normocytic anemia. Three consecutive blood cultures yield **coagulase-negative** *Staphylococcus epidermidis*; strain found to be **methicillin resistant**.

Imaging　　CXR (PA view): suggestive of **pulmonary edema**. Echo: confirms presence of **prosthetic aortic valve dehiscence** leading to incompetence and poor left ventricular function.

Treatment　　High-dose parenteral antibiotics—vancomycin (drug of choice for methicillin-resistant *S. aureus*), gentamicin, and oral rifampicin; surgical replacement of damaged prosthetic valve; prophylactic antibiotics (amoxicillin) for patients receiving oral/dental treatments to prevent transient bacteremia.

Discussion　　Prosthetic valve endocarditis is subdivided into two categories: early prosthetic valve endocarditis (EPVE), which becomes clinically manifest within 60 days after valve replacement (most commonly caused by *Staphylococcus epidermidis*, followed by gram-negative bacilli and *Candida*), and late prosthetic valve endocarditis (LPVE), which is manifested clinically more than 60 days after valve replacement (most commonly caused by viridans streptococci).

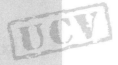
ID/CC   A 35-year-old male presents with high **fever**, malaise, headache, and a **hacking cough productive** of a small amount of mucoid sputum.

HPI   He has two **pet parrots** at home who have recently shown **signs of illness**.

PE   VS: fever; **bradycardia**. PE: auscultation of chest reveals **crepitant rales** over both lower lung fields; **splenomegaly** with mild hepatomegaly noted; multiple erythematous macules seen on face ("HORDER'S SPOTS").

Labs   Greater than fourfold rise in complement-fixing antibody titer to a group antigen suggestive of infection with *Chlamydia psittaci*; definitive diagnosis of psittacosis was made from sputum by isolation of *C. psittaci* in pretreated tissue culture cells.

Imaging   CXR, PA: **interstitial** patchy, bilateral **infiltrates**.

Gross Pathology   Principal lesions found in lungs, liver, and spleen.

Micro Pathology   Pulmonary lesion is an **interstitial pneumonitis**; mononuclear cells with ballooned cytoplasm containing inclusion bodies are observed. In the liver, focal necrosis of hepatocyte occurs along with Kupffer cell hyperplasia.

Treatment   Doxycycline; macrolides such as azithromycin are effective alternatives.

Discussion   Psittacosis is an acute infection caused by *Chlamydia psittaci*; it is characterized primarily by pneumonitis and systemic manifestations and is **transmitted** to humans by a variety of avian species, **principally psittacine birds (parrots, parakeets)**. A history of contact with birds, particularly sick birds, or of employment in a pet shop or in the poultry industry provides a clue to the diagnosis of psittacosis in a patient with pneumonia, especially if bradycardia and splenomegaly are also present.

TOP SECRET

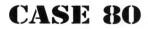
ID/CC
A 28-year-old black woman who is in her 27th week of pregnancy complains of **right flank pain, high-grade fever**, malaise, headache, and **dysuria.**

HPI
Thus far her pregnancy has been uneventful.

PE
VS: fever. PE: no peripheral edema; **right costovertebral angle tenderness; acutely painful fist percussion on right lumbar area** (POSITIVE GIORDANO'S SIGN).

Labs
CBC: leukocytosis with neutrophilia. UA: proteinuria; hematuria; abundant WBCs and **WBC casts**; pyocytes on sediment; alkaline pH; **urine culture > 100,000 colonies** of *Escherichia coli.*

Imaging
US, renal: slightly enlarged kidney.

Gross Pathology
Kidney enlarged, edematous, and hyperemic with microabscesses in medulla.

Micro Pathology
Pyocytes in tubules; **light blue neutrophils on supravital stain** (GLITTER CELLS); PMN infiltration of interstitium.

Treatment
Antibiotics according to sensitivity; ampicillin; in nonpregnant patients, fluoroquinolone or ampicillin and an aminoglycoside constitute initial treatment.

Discussion
An acute bacterial kidney infection caused mainly by gram-negative bacteria such as *E. coli, Klebsiella, Proteus, and Enterobacter*, acute pyelonephritis usually results from upward dissemination of lower urinary tract bacteria.

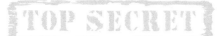

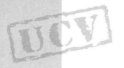
ID/CC

A 54-year-old **female** being treated in the ER is noted to have developed **progressively worsening abdominal pain and high-grade fever with chills.**

HPI

She presented to the ER a few hours ago with colicky abdominal pain and was diagnosed with **choledocholithiasis.**

PE

VS: **fever** (39.5°C), **hypotension** (BP 80/60); **tachycardia** (HR 120). PE: toxic-looking; **icteric**; abdominal exam reveals extremely **tender RUQ with hepatomegaly.**

Labs

CBC: leukocytosis with neutrophilia. LFTs: **markedly elevated bilirubin, AST, ALT, alkaline phosphatase and GGT.** Blood cultures grew *Escherichia coli.*

Imaging

CT, abdomen: **multiple hepatic abscesses**; distended gallbladder with perihepatic and pericholecystic fluid collections.

Treatment

Prolonged IV antibiotic therapy; emergent endoscopic (ERCP) or surgical biliary decompression; surgical **drainage** of the **abscesses** if no response to IV antibiotics.

Discussion

A **pyogenic liver abscess** is a pus-filled cavity within the liver caused by a bacterial infection, typically polymicrobial. The causes of liver abscess include **abdominal infection** such as appendicitis, diverticulitis, or perforated bowel; **sepsis; biliary tract infection**; or **liver trauma** leading to secondary infection. The most common bacteria involved are *E. coli, Klebsiella* **spp.**, *Enterococcus, Staphylococcus* **spp.**, *Streptococcus* **spp.**, and *Bacteroides.* Positive blood cultures are found in about half of patients with a pyogenic liver abscess and sepsis is a life-threatening complication. There is significant mortality even in treated patients and mortality is higher in those with multiple abscesses.

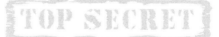

ID/CC   A 30-year-old **dairy farm worker** presents with complaints of **fever, headache, cough, pleuritic chest pain**, and malaise.

HPI   His work at the dairy involves **milking cows** and **looking after parturient cattle.**

PE   VS: fever; tachypnea. PE: mild icterus; bilateral **crackles** on chest auscultation.

Labs   CBC: normal WBC count. Mild elevation of serum bilirubin and liver enzymes; greater than fourfold increase in **complement-fixing antibody (against *Coxiella burnetii*)** titer between acute and convalescent sera (IFA technique for early detection of specific IgM Ab is the serodiagnostic method of choice); **negative Weil-Felix reaction**; *C. burnetii* isolated from sputum by inoculation of cultured human fetal diploid fibroblasts.

Imaging   CXR: right upper lobe **rounded opacity** that increased in size over a few days and cleared completely with treatment.

Treatment   **Doxycycline** is the first-line agent of therapy; fluoroquinolones and macrolides are effective alternatives (erythromycin can also be used).

Discussion   Q fever is caused by the rickettsia-like organism *Coxiella burnetii* and produces the clinical picture of primary atypical pneumonia. Q fever differs from the other human rickettsioses in that rash is absent and **transmission** is usually **by the airborne route**. *C. burnetii* localizes in the **mammary glands and uterus of pregnant cattle**, sheep, and goats, in which infection is mild or inapparent; **infected placentas, postpartum discharges, and the feces of these animals** are the **principal sources of contaminated material** in the environment. Humans acquire Q fever by inhaling aerosolized particles from such substances; particularly **at risk** are **dairy and slaughterhouse workers**.

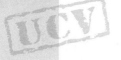

CASE 83

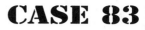

BACTERIOLOGY

ID/CC A 27-year-old male **researcher** presents with sudden-onset **fever**, chills, headache, a **skin rash**, and **painful** swelling of multiple limb **joints**.

HPI Careful history reveals that he was **bitten by a rat** in his laboratory a few days ago; the bite wound has now healed.

PE VS: **fever**. PE: morbilliform **rash** noted over extremities, particularly the hands and feet; **painful swelling** and restriction of movement noted over **both wrist and knee joints**.

Labs CBC: leukocytosis. *Streptobacillus moniliformis* isolated from blood and synovial fluid of inflamed joints; agglutinins to *S. moniliformis* demonstrated in significant titers.

Treatment Amoxicillin/clavulonic acid (**doxycycline** can also be used).

Discussion Rat bite fever, which is caused by *Streptobacillus moniliformis*, is an acute febrile illness that is usually accompanied by a skin rash; **most cases result from the bites of wild or lab rats**, although mice, squirrels, weasels, dogs, and cats may also transmit the disease by bites or scratches. The disease is called **Haverhill fever** when *S. moniliformis* is transmitted by drinking rat-excrement-contaminated milk. Distribution is probably worldwide, with most cases occurring in crowded cities characterized by poor sanitation.

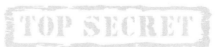

ID/CC   A 30-year-old male who lives in the **western part of the United States** presents with **high fever**, shaking **chills**, severe headache, myalgias, and diarrhea.

HPI   He reports having had **similar symptoms 10 days ago** that lasted for 4 to 5 days, followed by defervescence accompanied by drenching sweats and marked prostration. He had been **hiking in a tick-infested forest** until about a week before the development of symptoms.

PE   VS: **fever**.

Labs   **Spirochetes found on thick smears of peripheral blood** obtained during febrile period and **stained with Wright or Giemsa stain**.

Treatment   **Doxycycline** is the drug of choice (erythromycin may also be used).

Discussion   Relapsing fever is an **acute louse-borne or tick-borne infection** that is caused by blood spirochetes of the genus *Borrelia*; it is characterized by **recurrent febrile episodes separated by asymptomatic intervals**. Unlike other spirochetes, the etiologic agent can readily be detected with Giemsa stain or Wright's stain. *B. recurrentis* is the **cause of louse-borne relapsing fever**, whereas a variety of different species produce the **tick-borne disease**. In the United States, the predominant species are *B. hermsii* and *B. turicatae*. Most patients experience the Jarisch–Herxheimer reaction within the first 2 hours of treatment.

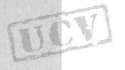

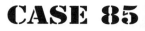

CASE 85

BACTERIOLOGY

ID/CC	A 6-year-old male presents with fever, intense headache, myalgia, dry cough, and a **rash that began peripherally** (on his wrists and ankles) but now involves the entire body, **including the palms and soles.**
HPI	The child lives in North Carolina and indicates that he was **bitten by an insect** a few weeks ago while playing in the woods near his home.
PE	VS: fever. PE: lethargy; ill appearance; **petechial rash** all over body, including palms and soles.
Labs	CBC: thrombocytopenia; prolonged bleeding and clotting time. Positive Hess capillary test (RUMPEL-LEEDE PHENOMENON). UA: proteinuria; hematuria. *Rickettsia rickettsii* detected on immunohistologic staining of skin rash biopsy.
Gross Pathology	Hemorrhagic necrosis in brain and kidneys; nodular formation in glia.
Micro Pathology	Inflammatory lymphocytic and plasma cell perivascular infiltration; endothelial edema with abundant rickettsiae; microthrombus formation **with necrotic vasculitis.**
Treatment	**Doxycycline** or **chloramphenicol.**
Discussion	*Rickettsia rickettsii* is the causative organism of Rocky Mountain spotted fever; *Dermacentor*, **a wood tick, is the vector.** The organism's tropism for endothelial cells results in vasculitis, edema, thrombosis, and ischemia. Ironically, Rocky Mountain spotted fever is endemic to the East Coast of the United States.

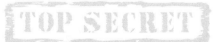

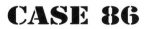

CASE 86

ID/CC   A 30-year-old male presents with sudden-onset, crampy **abdominal pain and diarrhea**.

HPI   The diarrhea is **watery** and contains **mucus**. The patient also complains of low-grade fever with chills, malaise, nausea, and vomiting. Careful history reveals that he had ingested **partially cooked eggs** at a poultry farm 24 hours before his symptoms began.

PE   VS: fever; tachycardia. PE: mild diffuse abdominal tenderness; mild dehydration.

Labs   Stool culture yields *Salmonella typhimurium*; stained stool demonstrates PMNs.

Gross Pathology   Intestinal mucosal erythema (limited to the colon) and some superficial ulcers.

Micro Pathology   Mixed inflammatory infiltrate in mucosa; superficial epithelial erosions.

Treatment   Fluid and electrolyte replacement therapy; **antibiotics withheld**, as they **prolong carrier state**. Antibiotic therapy only for malnourished, severely ill, bacteremic, and sickle cell disease patients.

Discussion   Salmonella infection is acquired through the ingestion of food (**eggs, meat, poultry**) or water contaminated with animal or human feces; individuals with **low gastric acidity** are also susceptible.

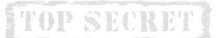

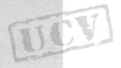

BACTERIOLOGY

ID/CC
A 14-year-old male who is known to have **sickle cell anemia** presents with throbbing **pain, redness,** and **swelling** of the **right thigh.**

HPI
The patient also complains of fever and chills of 1 week's duration. He has a few **pet turtles** at home.

PE
VS: **fever**; tachycardia. PE: pallor; redness, swelling, and tenderness over right thigh; effusion demonstrated in right knee joint; limitation of range of motion of right knee.

Labs
CBC: leukocytosis; elevated ESR. PBS: irreversible **sickling**; blood culture reveals *Salmonella typhimurium* (most common); organism also isolated from pus aspirated from right femur (diagnostic of **osteomyelitis**).

Imaging
Nuc: **increased uptake in metaphyseal region** of right femur. XR (usually normal during the first 10 days of illness) may reveal changes of bone resorption, detached necrotic cortical bone (SEQUESTRUM), and laminated periosteal new-bone formation (INVOLUCRUM).

Gross Pathology
Dense, pale, sclerotic-appearing area in shaft.

Micro Pathology
Changes include suppurative and ischemic destructive necrosis, fibrosis, and ultimate bone repair.

Treatment
Parenteral antibiotics, with **fluoroquinolones** being first-line agents (**third-generation cephalosporins** may also be used).

Discussion
A striking association has been noted between diseases producing hemolysis (e.g., sickle cell anemia, malaria, and bartonellosis) and salmonella infections; elderly patients with impaired host defense mechanisms, those with hepatosplenic schistosomiasis, and AIDS patients are also at increased risk of severe and recurrent salmonella bacteremia. Salmonella osteomyelitis in sickle cell patients presents primarily in young individuals and typically affects long bones. It is believed that the functional asplenic state found in most sickle cell patients contributes to the increased prevalence of salmonella osteomyelitis.

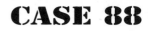

ID/CC   A **2-month-old** female infant presents with extensive **bullae** and large areas of denuded skin.

HPI   Her mother had suffered from **staphylococcal mastitis** 1 week ago.

PE   VS: fever. PE: large areas of red, painful, denuded skin on periorbital and peribuccal areas; flaccid bullae with **easy dislodgment of epidermis under pressure** (NIKOLSKY'S SIGN); mucosal surfaces largely uninvolved.

Labs   Vesicle fluid sterile; *Staphylococcus aureus* on blood culture.

Treatment   IV penicillinase-resistant penicillin (e.g., nafcillin, oxacillin). Treat with erythromycin if patient is allergic to penicillin.

Discussion   Scalded skin syndrome is caused by the exfoliating effect of **staphylococcal exotoxin**. The action of the exotoxin is to degrade desmoglein in desmosomes in the skin.

ID/CC   A 10-year-old white female complains of difficulty swallowing, pain in both ears, and fever of 1 week's duration; she also complains of an extensive skin rash.

HPI   The child is fully immunized and has been well until now.

PE   VS: fever. PE: **extensive erythematous rash** ("GOOSE-PIMPLE SUNBURN") on neck, groin, and axillae; desquamation and **peeling of fingertips**; circumoral pallor; **lines of hyperpigmentation with tiny petechiae** (PASTIA'S SIGN) in antecubital fossae; **bright red lingual papillae superimposed on white coat** ("STRAWBERRY TONGUE"); pharyngitis with exudative tonsillitis; cervical lymphadenopathy; normal eardrums.

Labs   CBC: leukocytosis with neutrophilia. **Group A β-hemolytic** *Streptococcus pyogenes* on throat swab and culture.

Micro Pathology   Toxin-induced vasodilation; inflammatory polymorphonuclear epidermal infiltrate; interstitial nephritis; lymph node hyperplasia.

Treatment   Penicillin; erythromycin.

Discussion   Scarlet fever is a streptococcal infection that is characterized by **morbilliform rash** due to **hypersensitivity to erythrogenic toxin** Complications include otitis media, pneumonia, glomerulonephritis, osteomyelitis, and rheumatic fever.

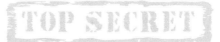

ID/CC   A 21-year-old female college student complains of low-grade fever along with **pain** and **swelling** in the left knee of 5 days' duration.

HPI   She had been to her family physician 2 weeks ago because of **dysuria** and a **purulent vaginal discharge** (due to gonococcal infection) and was given an "antibiotic shot." She was asymptomatic until 4 days ago. She then developed **fever, chills**, and pain in both wrists and in her left ankle, which disappeared when the pain appeared in her left knee (MIGRATORY POLYARTHRALGIA).

PE   Swollen, **tender, warm** left knee with **limited range of motion**; white vaginal discharge.

Labs   Intracellular, **bean-shaped gram-negative diplococci** (GONOCOCCI) and **markedly elevated WBC count** on urethral smear and **synovial fluid aspirate** culture of synovial aspirate grows gonococci.

Imaging   XR, knee: soft tissue swelling.

Treatment   IV ceftriaxone.

Discussion   Almost always accompanied by synovitis and effusion, gonococcal arthritis can rapidly destroy articular cartilage and may be associated with skin rash and C5, C6, C7, and C8 complement deficiencies. Single joints are usually affected, most often the wrists, fingers, knees, and ankles.

BACTERIOLOGY

ID/CC   A 36-year-old male executive comes to the emergency room because of the development of **sudden nausea, vomiting, and diarrhea** with **blood and mucus** (dysentery) as well as crampy abdominal pain for 2 days.

HPI   He had just returned from a business trip in **South America**.

PE   VS: low-grade fever. PE: mild dehydration; hyperactive bowel sounds; tender abdomen without definite peritoneal irritation.

Labs   **Leukocytes on stool examination**; *Shigella* isolated on stool culture; on microbiology, organism does not ferment lactose and is **not motile**.

Micro Pathology   Colitis evidenced by severe neutrophilic and mononuclear cell infiltration of lamina propria; ulcers; mucus depletion.

Treatment   Rehydration with antibiotic therapy (TMP-SMX or fluoroquinolone).

Discussion   Shigellosis outbreaks occur primarily in areas with **overcrowding** and **poor hygiene** (fecal-oral transmission); **arthritis, conjunctivitis, and urethritis** (REITER'S SYNDROME) may be complications in HLA-B27-positive individuals. Like *Salmonella, Shigella* causes bloody diarrhea by invading the intestinal mucosa, causing intestinal ulceration and inflammation.

ID/CC

A 56-year-old hospitalized male is found to have an abrupt-onset **high-grade fever** with chills a few hours after he underwent nephrolithotomy.

HPI

He was diagnosed with chronic nephrolithiasis with **recurrent UTIs**; a surgery intern also noted **poor urine output**.

PE

VS: fever; tachycardia; **hypotension**; tachypnea. PE: confused and disoriented; hyperventilating; diaphoresis; **hands warm** and pink with rapid capillary refill; pulse bounding; on chest auscultation, air entry found to be bilaterally reduced.

Labs

CBC: **leukocytosis** with left shift; neutrophils contain **toxic granulations, Döhle bodies**, and cytoplasmic vacuoles; band forms > 10%; thrombocytopenia. Prolongation of thrombin time, decreased fibrinogen, and presence of D-dimers (suggesting DIC); raised BUN and creatinine. ABGs: metabolic acidosis (increased anion gap due to lactic acidosis) and hypoxemia (due to **ARDS**). Blood and urine **culture yields** *Escherichia coli*.

Imaging

CXR: evidence of noncardiogenic pulmonary edema (ARDS).

Treatment

IV antibiotics (with adequate gram-negative coverage); supportive management of multiorgan failure (azotemia, ARDS, and DIC); recombinant human activated protein C for high-risk cases.

Discussion

Almost any bacterium can cause a bacteremia, including *E. coli* (most common), *Klebsiella, Proteus, Pseudomonas* (associated with antibiotic therapy and burn wounds), *Bacteroides fragilis* (causes of anaerobic septicemias), *Staphylococcus aureus, Streptococcus pneumoniae*, and pediatric septicemia due to *E. coli* and *Streptococcus agalactiae*. Gram-negative bacteria release endotoxins; the release of endotoxin into the circulation leads to the activation of macrophages and monocytes, which in turn release cytokines. These cytokines trigger cascade reactions that lead to the clinical and biochemical manifestations of the sepsis syndrome.

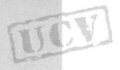

CASE 93

ID/CC
A 50-year-old alcoholic white male presents with **fever, abdominal pain**, and rapidly progressive distention of the abdomen.

HPI
He was diagnosed with **alcoholic cirrhosis** 1 month ago, when he was admitted to the hospital with jaundice and hematemesis.

PE
VS: fever. PE: icterus; on palpation, abdominal tenderness with guarding; fluid thrill and shifting dullness to percussion (due to **ascites**); **splenomegaly**; decreased bowel sounds.

Labs
CBC: **leukocytosis**. Ascitic fluid leukocyte count > 500/cc; PMNs (350/cc) elevated; ascitic proteins and glucose depressed; gram-negative bacilli in ascitic fluid; *Escherichia coli* isolated in culture; elevated AST and ALT (AST > ALT).

Imaging
KUB: ground-glass haziness (due to ascites); no evidence of free air. US, abdomen: cirrhotic shrunken liver; **ascites; splenomegaly; increased portal vein diameter and flow.** EGD: esophageal varices.

Gross Pathology
Fibrinopurulent exudate covering surface of peritoneum; fibrosis may lead to formation of adhesions.

Micro Pathology
PMNs and fibrin on serosal surfaces in various stages with presence of granulation tissue and fibrosis.

Treatment
Treat empirically with a third-generation cephalosporin such as cefotaxime followed by culture sensitivity–guided therapy; long-term prophylaxis with fluoroquinolones may be needed following treatment; supportive treatment for cirrhosis.

Discussion
The spontaneous or primary form of peritonitis occurs in patients with advanced chronic liver disease and concomitant ascites; *E. coli* is the most common cause of secondary peritonitis.

TOP SECRET

ID/CC A 25-year-old female complains of low-grade fever and myalgia of 3 weeks' duration.

HPI She has a history of **rheumatic heart disease** (RHD). One month ago, she underwent a **dental extraction** and did not take the antibiotics that were prescribed for her.

PE VS: fever. PE: pallor; small peripheral hemorrhages with slight nodular character (JANEWAY LESIONS); small, tender nodules on finger and toe pads (OSLER'S NODES); subungual linear streaks (SPLINTER HEMORRHAGES); petechial hemorrhages on conjunctiva, oral mucosa, and upper extremities; mild splenomegaly; apical diastolic murmur on cardiovascular exam; fundus exam shows oval retinal hemorrhages (ROTH'S SPOTS).

Labs CBC/PBS: normocytic, normochromic anemia. UA: microscopic hematuria. Growth of penicillin-sensitive *Streptococcus viridans* on five of six blood cultures.

Imaging Echo: vegetations along atrial surface of **mitral valve**.

Gross Pathology Embolism from vegetative growths on valves may embolize peripherally (left-sided) or to the lung (right-sided).

Micro Pathology Bacteria form nidus of infection in previously scarred or damaged valves; bacteria divide unimpeded once infection takes hold with further deposition of fibrin and platelets; peripheral symptoms such as Osler's nodes are believed to result from deposition of immune complexes.

Treatment IV β-lactamase-resistant penicillin and gentamicin; bacteriostatic treatments ineffective.

Discussion *S. viridans* is the most common cause of subacute infective endocarditis, while *Staphylococcus aureus* is the most common cause of acute bacterial endocarditis. Prophylactic antibiotics should be given to all RHD patients before any dental procedure. The disease continues to be associated with a high mortality rate.

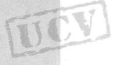

CASE 95

ID/CC   A 54-year-old white female complains of **spiking fever**, chills, **loss of appetite**, several bouts of diarrhea, and **right upper quadrant pain**.

HPI   **Ten days ago** she underwent an apparently uncomplicated emergency **surgery for suppurative cholecystitis** and was subsequently discharged and sent home.

PE   VS: fever. PE: pallor; slight icterus; **pain on percussion of right costal region**; well-healed surgical wound with no evidence of infection; liver not palpable; crepitant rales on right lung base.

Labs   CBC: **elevated WBC count (17,000) with predominance of neutrophils.**

Imaging   CXR: elevated right hemidiaphragm; slight right pleural effusion. US/CT: **complex fluid collection below diaphragm.**

Treatment   Percutaneous drainage under ultrasonic or fluoroscopic guidance followed by regular blood and radiologic exams; surgical exploration and drainage.

Discussion   Subdiaphragmatic abscess most commonly occurs after abdominal surgery, mainly with septic, emergency procedures; it typically presents 1 week or more postoperatively.

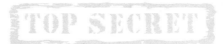

ID/CC A 6-week-old male, the son of a **prostitute**, is brought to the family doctor because of persistent, sometimes **bloody mucopurulent nasal discharge, anal ulcers**, and a generalized **rash**.

HPI The child was delivered at home, and the mother did not receive any prenatal care.

PE Weak-looking, **icteric** infant with hoarse cry; does not move right limb (**pseudoparalysis**); bloody purulent discharge evident at nares; generalized lymphadenopathy; hepatosplenomegaly; **maculopapular rash** with desquamation on back and buttocks; **bullae on hands and feet**.

Labs CBC: anemia. **VDRL** in both mother and child **positive**; direct hyperbilirubinemia; negative Coombs' test; *Treponema pallidum* seen on nasal exudate.

Imaging XR, plain: periostitis of long bones; bilateral moth-eaten lesions; focal defect in proximal tibial epiphysis with increased density of epiphyseal line (WIMBERGER'S SIGN).

Gross Pathology Pathologic features seen if neonatal disease is left untreated include syphilitic chondritis and rhinitis (causes **saddle-nose deformity**), pathologic fractures, **bowing of the tibia** (SABER SHIN), **V-shaped incisors** (HUTCHINSON'S TEETH), multicuspid molars (MULBERRY MOLARS), interstitial keratitis, and deafness.

Treatment Penicillin.

Discussion *Treponema pallidum* is a spirochete; in utero vertical transmission occurs from an infected mother to the fetus. Congenital syphilis occurs maximally during 16 to 36 weeks of gestation and may be the cause of stillbirth. It is preventable if the mother has received adequate treatment.

CASE 97

BACTERIOLOGY

ID/CC   An 18-year-old white male presents with a **painless ulcer** on his **penis**.

HPI   He admits to having had **unprotected intercourse** with a prostitute 3 weeks ago.

PE   **Painless, single, rounded, firm papule with well-defined margins on dorsal aspect of glans penis that ulcerates** ("HARD CHANCRE"); nontender, rubbery bilateral inguinal lymphadenopathy.

Labs   Treponemes on **dark-field examination** of exudate from chancre; VDRL positive; **FTA-ABS positive**; ELISA for HIV negative.

Micro Pathology   Capillary dilatation with plasma cell, PMN, and macrophage infiltration; fibroblastic reaction.

Treatment   **Benzathine penicillin G** IM, 2.4 MU single dose.

Discussion   An STD caused by *Treponema pallidum*, a spirochete, primary syphilis is characterized by the appearance of a painless chancre in the area of inoculation. If left untreated, secondary and tertiary syphilis may ensue. Other STDs, such as AIDS, are more prevalent in patients with syphilis

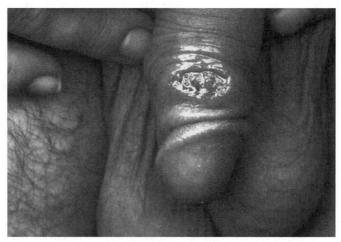

Figure 097 Well-demarcated "punched out" painless ulcer on underside of foreskin (chancre).

ID/CC   A 23-year-old female presents with a **nonpruritic skin eruption, hair loss,** and generalized fatigue and weakness.

HPI   She admits to having had **multiple sexual partners** and **unprotected sex.** She has had two spontaneous abortions.

PE   Extensive **raised, copper-colored, maculopapular, desquamative rash on palms and soles**; generalized nontender **lymphadenopathy** with hepatosplenomegaly; large, pale, **coalescent, flat-topped papules and plaques** in groin (CONDYLOMATA LATA); dull, erythematous **mucous patches in mouth**; hair loss (ALOPECIA) in tail of eyebrows.

Labs   Skin lesions, mucous patches in mouth, and condylomata lata positive for **treponemes; positive VDRL; positive FTA-ABS;** ELISA negative for HIV; CSF VDRL negative.

Treatment   IM benzathine **penicillin G.**

Discussion   **Sexual partners must be treated.**

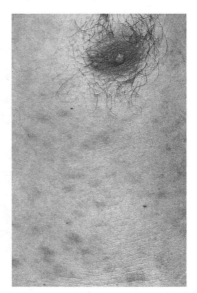

Figure 098 Diffuse macular rash on the trunk.

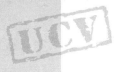

CASE 99

ID/CC A 54-year-old man presents with **ataxia, mental status changes**, grossly **deformed ankle joints**, and **shooting pains** in his extremities.

HPI He remembers having had a "boil" on his penis (PRIMARY SYPHILITIC CHANCRE) many years ago that went away by itself. He also recalls having had a scaling rash on the soles of his feet and the palms of his hands (due to secondary syphilis) some time ago.

PE Painless **subcutaneous granulomatous nodules** (GUMMAS); **reduced joint position and vibration sense in both lower extremities** (due to bilateral dorsal column destruction); loss of deep tendon reflexes in both lower limbs; loss of pain sensation and **deformed ankle and knee joints with effusion** (CHARCOT'S NEUROPATHIC ARTHROPATHY); **broad-based gait**; positive Romberg's sign (due to sensory ataxia); **pupillary light reflex lost but accommodation reflex retained** (ARGYLL ROBERTSON PUPILS).

Labs Positive VDRL and *Treponema pallidum* hemagglutination assay (TP-HA). **LP: pleocytosis and increased proteins in CSF**; VDRL positive. Normal blood glucose levels.

Imaging CXR: **"tree-bark calcification"** of ascending aorta.

Gross Pathology Obliterative endarteritis and meningoencephalitis.

Micro Pathology Proliferation of microglia; demyelinization and axonal loss in dorsal roots and columns.

Treatment Penicillin.

Discussion **Tabes dorsalis** usually develops 15 to 20 years after initial infection. There may also be visceral involvement (can cause neurogenic bladder).

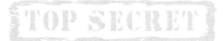

ID/CC   A 12-year-old white male presents with **stiffness of the jaw** and neck along with inability to swallow.

HPI   Twelve days ago he stepped on a **rusty nail**, which produced a small **puncture wound**; the area is now red, hard, and swollen with pus. He has been experiencing tingling sensations and spasms in his calf muscles. He has not received any immunizations within the past 10 years.

PE   **Jaw muscle rigidity** (TRISMUS); **facial muscle spasm** (RISUS SARDONICUS); **dysphagia; neck rigidity**; normal deep tendon reflexes; profuse sweating; patient alert, apprehensive, restless, and hyperactive during PE; loud noise elicits **painful spasms** of face, neck, abdomen, and back, the latter producing **opisthotonos**.

Labs   CBC, CSF, blood chemistries normal.

Gross Pathology   There may be fractures of ribs or vertebrae with sustained spasms.

Treatment   **Surgical debridement of wound**; tetanus immune globulin intramuscularly or intrathecally; diazepam; phenobarbital; tetanus toxoid; penicillin IV.

Discussion   Tetanus is caused by **tetanospasmin**, a neurotoxin produced by *Clostridium tetani*, an obligate anaerobic, spore-forming, gram-positive rod; the toxin blocks the release of the inhibitory neurotransmitter glycine in the anterior horn cells. Tetanus often occurs in IV drug abusers; neonates of nonimmunized mothers may become infected through the **umbilical cord stump**. The disease may occur even **years** after injury or infection and may also involve the autonomic nervous system (arrhythmias, high/low blood pressure).

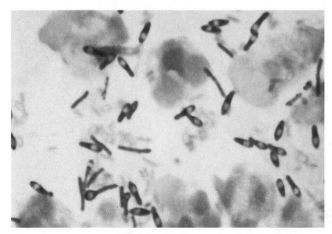

Figure 100 Gram-positive rods with oval subterminal and terminal spores.

ID/CC A 15-day-old **infant** is brought by his mother to the pediatric emergency room in a state of marked **muscle rigidity and spasm**.

HPI The mother is illiterate and did **not receive any prenatal care**; the delivery was conducted at home and, according to her, was uneventful and full term. The child did **not receive any immunizations**; directed questioning reveals that he has been crying excessively for the past 2 weeks and has not been feeding normally.

PE Extremely ill-looking infant in a state of **generalized rigidity and opisthotonus**; on slightest touch or noise, spasm worsens and he develops a stridor and becomes cyanosed.

Labs Diagnosis is largely clinical; **culture of umbilical stump yields** *Clostridium tetani.*

Treatment **Ventilatory assistance**; **supportive** management; maintenance of nutritional, fluid, and electrolyte balance; **human tetanus immunoglobulin** for neutralizing unbound toxin; antibiotics such as **penicillin** or **metronidazole** to stop toxin production by killing the organism; control of tetanic spasms with diazepam.

Discussion Tetanus neonatorum accounts for a considerable proportion of infant deaths in developing countries, primarily owing to the **lack of availability of good prenatal care** (no tetanus immunization); untrained birth attendants in rural areas use **contaminated** material to cut or anoint the **umbilical cord**. Tetanus is caused by *Clostridium tetani*, a grampositive, motile, nonencapsulated, anaerobic, spore-bearing bacillus; its effects are mediated through production of a powerful **neurotoxin** (**tetanospasmin**). The toxin acts principally on the spinal cord, altering normal control of the reflex arc by suppressing the inhibition regularly mediated by the internuncial neurons.

ID/CC   A 30-year-old **woman** presents to the ER with an abrupt-onset **high fever, vomiting, profuse diarrhea**, severe muscle aches, and disorientation.

HPI   One day ago she developed an **extensive skin rash** all over her body. Her husband says she used a **vaginal sponge** for contraception.

PE   VS: fever; tachycardia; hypotension. PE: extremely toxic-looking; drowsy but responding to verbal commands; **extensive scarlatiniform rash** seen involving entire body; pharyngeal, conjunctival, and vaginal mucosa congested (frank hyperemia); no neck rigidity or Kernig's sign demonstrable; funduscopic exam normal; no localizing neurologic deficits.

Labs   CBC: leukocytosis; thrombocytopenia. UA: mild pyuria (in absence of UTI). BUN and creatinine elevated; blood cultures sterile; **culture of cervical secretions grows *Staphylococcus aureus***. LP: CSF normal. Serology for Rocky Mountain spotted fever, leptospirosis, and measles negative.

Treatment   **Vigorous IV fluids** and parenteral **penicillinase-resistant penicillin** or first-generation cephalosporins; patient in this case recovered, and typical skin desquamation was seen over palms and soles during convalescence.

Discussion   Toxic shock syndrome results from infection with *Staphylococcus aureus*. Its effects are mediated through the **exotoxin TSST-1**, which functions as a superantigen, stimulating the production of interleukin-1 and tumor necrosis factor. Staphylococcal TSS has been associated with the use of **vaginal contraceptive sponges** and with many types of localized staphylococcal soft tissue infections. Most cases of TSS occur in **menstruating women**.

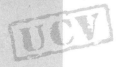

CASE 103

ID/CC   A 25-year-old male U.S. citizen on **vacation in Mexico** presents with abrupt-onset explosive **watery diarrhea, abdominal cramps**, and a **low-grade fever** and chills.

HPI   The patient does not complain of tenesmus or passage of blood or mucus in his stools, but he does complain of a feeling of **urgency** to defecate.

PE   VS: low-grade fever. PE: unremarkable.

Labs   No erythrocytes, WBCs, or parasites seen in stained stool; bioassays for enterotoxigenic *Escherichia coli* (**ETEC**) reveal presence of the labile **enterotoxin (LT)** (tests available only for research purposes).

Treatment Fluid replacement; antibiotics (fluoroquinolone or TMP-SMX) with loperamide; prevention with careful hygienic practices and prophylactic fluoroquinolone or bismuth subsalicylate with loperamide.

Discussion Traveler's diarrhea is a self-limited condition that develops within 1 to 2 days of ingestion of contaminated food or drinks. Over three-fourths of cases of traveler's diarrhea are caused by bacteria, with enterotoxigenic *E. coli* the most frequent cause (may also be caused by enteropathogenic *E. coli* and, in Mexico, by an enteroadherent *E. coli*). Other common pathogens include *Shigella* species, *Campylobacter jejuni, Aeromonas* species, *Plesiomonas shigelloides, Salmonella* species, and noncholera vibrios. Rotavirus and Norwalk agent are the most common viral causes; *Giardia, Cryptosporidium*, and, rarely, *Entamoeba histolytica* are parasitic pathogens. Enterotoxigenic *E. coli* produce enterotoxins that bind to intestinal receptors and **activate adenyl cyclase** in the intestinal cell to produce an increase in the level of the cyclic nucleotides cAMP (LT, labile toxin) and cGMP (ST, stable toxin), which markedly augments sodium, chloride, and water loss, thereby producing a **secretory diarrhea**.

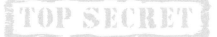

ID/CC A 6-year-old male is brought to the ER in a delirious state with fever and marked dyspnea that have rapidly progressed over the past 2 days.

HPI His mother, an Asian immigrant, was diagnosed and treated for pulmonary tuberculosis a few months ago. He has had a low-grade fever, cough, malaise, and night sweats for the past 2 months. The child has not received prophylactic isoniazid or BCG vaccination.

PE VS: fever; tachycardia; marked tachypnea; hypotension. PE: toxic and stuporous; pallor; central cyanosis; extensive rales and rhonchi bilaterally; hepatosplenomegaly; lymphadenopathy; funduscopy reveals choroidal tubercles.

Labs CBC: lymphocytosis; normochromic, normocytic anemia. Increased ESR; Mantoux skin test negative (false negative may occur during incubation and with severe disease); staining and culture of transbronchial and bone marrow biopsy specimens reveal presence of *Mycobacterium tuberculosis*; PCR for tuberculosis positive; ELISA for HIV negative.

Imaging CXR: soft, uniformly distributed fine nodules throughout both lung fields (MILIARY MOTTLING).

Gross Pathology Myriad 1- to 2-mm granulomas demonstrable in lungs, liver, and bone marrow biopsy specimens.

Micro Pathology Granulomas with central caseous necrosis surrounded by epithelial cells, Langerhan's cells, lymphocytes, plasma cells, and fibroblasts in affected tissues.

Treatment Multidrug antitubercular therapy with isoniazid, rifampicin, pyrazinamide, and ethambutol or streptomycin; steroids may be indicated.

Discussion Miliary tuberculosis results from widespread hematogenous dissemination and often presents with a perplexing fever, dyspnea, anemia, and splenomegaly; the disease is more fulminant in children than in adults.

BACTERIOLOGY

ID/CC   A 14-year-old male immigrant complains of malaise, **weight loss, fever, and night sweats** of 6 weeks' duration; he also has a mild cough that began to produce **bloody sputum** 3 days prior to his admission.

HPI   The patient's **mother** has been diagnosed with pulmonary **tuberculosis** and is currently receiving treatment for it.

PE   VS: mild fever. PE: **malnourished**; low height and weight for age; bronchial breath sounds with crepitant rales heard over right supramammary area.

Labs   CBC/PBS: normocytic, normochromic anemia; WBC count normal with relative **lymphocytosis. Increased ESR**; sputum stained with ZN stain **positive for acid-fast bacilli**; positive radiometric culture for *Mycobacterium tuberculosis*; positive ELISA for TB; positive **intradermal tuberculin injection** (MANTOUX TEST).

Imaging CXR: small cavity with streaky infiltrates in right upper lobe; hilar lymphadenopathy; calcified lung lesion (GHON'S LESION); Ghon's lesion and calcified lymph node (RANKE COMPLEX).

Gross Pathology **Primary tuberculosis** usually consists of **lesions in lower lung lobes** and in subpleural locations; cavitation rare; **secondary TB** or reinfection characterized by cavitary lesions usually located in **apical regions**.

Micro Pathology Multinucleated epithelioid **Langerhan's cells** surround core of **caseating necrosis** in lung parenchyma, producing fibroblastic reaction at periphery with lymphocytic infiltration and proliferation (TUBERCLE).

Treatment Multiple drug therapy with isoniazid (INH), rifampin, ethambutol, pyrazinamide, and/or streptomycin.

Discussion Pulmonary tuberculosis is caused by *Mycobacterium tuberculosis*, an acid-fast, gram-positive aerobic bacillus. An **increasing incidence in AIDS patients** has been observed; drug resistance is becoming common.

ID/CC	A 12-year-old white male is brought to his pediatrician because of an **ulcer** on his right wrist together with **swelling of the lymph nodes** in the right axillae with **suppuration**.
HPI	He had just returned from summer camp and, upon questioning, admits to having played with **rabbits** at the camp's breeding grounds. He has been suffering from **fever**, headache, and muscle aches for almost a week.
PE	VS: fever. PE: indurated erythematous nodule with ulcer formation on right wrist; right axillary adenopathy with pus formation; lymphangitis; mild splenomegaly; scattered rales in both lung bases.
Labs	CBC: **normal WBC count. Increased ESR**; elevated C-reactive protein; positive agglutination test; *Francisella tularensis* on direct fluorescent antibody staining of material from ulcer.
Imaging	CXR: bilateral basilar interstitial infiltrates.
Gross Pathology	Enlarged, indurated lymph nodes with necrosis and suppuration; skin nodule at site of inoculation with ulcer formation.
Micro Pathology	Necrosis and suppuration of lymph nodes; pulmonary and disseminated lesions; **granulomatous nodules** with central caseating necrosis.
Treatment	Streptomycin or tetracycline; surgical drainage of fluctuant lymph nodes.
Discussion	Tularemia is an acute zoonosis caused by *Francisella tularensis*, a non-motile, aerobic, gram-negative bacillus; it is transmitted through contact with rabbits, squirrels, or other rodents or tick bites. It may be ulcero-glandular, tonsillar, oculoglandular, pneumonitic, or typhoidal.

TOP SECRET

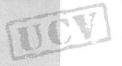
ID/CC   A 27-year-old male is admitted to the hospital for evaluation of **increasing fever** of unknown origin along with malaise, headache, sore throat, cough, and **constipation**.

HPI   He visited Southeast Asia 3 weeks ago but did not receive any prior vaccinations.

PE   VS: **bradycardia**; fever; **fever charting reveals "stepladder" pattern.** PE: mild hepatosplenomegaly; faint **erythematous macules seen over trunk** ("ROSE SPOTS").

Labs   CBC: neutropenia with relative lymphocytosis. **Widal's test** positive in significant titers; blood and stool cultures reveal *Salmonella typhi*.

Gross Pathology   **Infection of Peyer's patches** in terminal ileum leads to necrosis of underlying mucosa, producing longitudinal oval ulcerations.

Micro Pathology   Ulcers bordered by mononuclear cells; typhoid nodules with lymphocytes and macrophages may be present in liver, spleen, and lymph nodes.

Treatment   **Ciprofloxacin** or **third-generation cephalosporins**; steroids for severe infection.

Discussion   Because infection is acquired from contaminated food or water, typhoid vaccine is recommended for all those traveling to areas that have had typhoid epidemics. Three vaccines are available: the parenteral vaccine containing the capsular polysaccharide and the oral vaccine containing live attenuated organisms are more effective than the parenteral vaccine containing whole killed organisms. *S. typhi* is transmitted only by humans, whereas all other *Salmonella* species have an animal as well as a human reservoir.

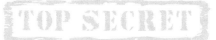

ID/CC　A 19-year-old male goes to his health clinic complaining of **painful urination and discharge**.

HPI　The patient had **casual sex with a classmate** while at a party **2 weeks ago**. He has had no previous STDs.

PE　Watery yellowish-green discharge from meatus; no penile ulcerations or inguinal lymphadenopathy.

Labs　**Numerous neutrophils but no bacteria** on Gram stain of discharge; **positive** direct immunofluorescence using monoclonal **antibody against** *Chlamydia*; routine bacterial cultures, including Thayer-Martin, do not show growth.

Treatment　Tetracycline; **doxycycline**; azithromycin; treat both patient and sexual partner.

Discussion　The most common cause of nongonococcal urethritis is *Chlamydia trachomatis*; less frequently it is caused by *Ureaplasma urealyticum*. It is frequently coincident with gonococcal urethritis.

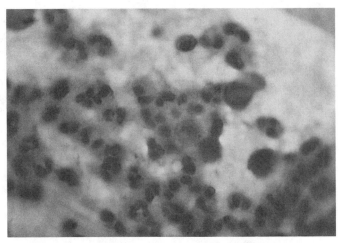

Figure 108 Gram stain of urethral discharge demonstrating numerous neutrophils.

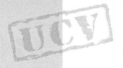

ID/CC   A 25-year-old **sexually active female** complains of **burning on urination.**

HPI   She also complains of pain in the lower abdomen and **increased frequency of urination.**

PE   Mild suprapubic tenderness.

Labs   UA: mild proteinuria; hematuria; WBCs but no casts seen. Urine culture reveals > 100,000 *Escherichia coli* organisms present.

Gross Pathology   Infection ascends the urinary tract (urethritis, cystitis, pyelonephritis); mucosal hyperemia and edema.

Micro Pathology   Urothelial hyperplasia and metaplasia.

Treatment   TMP-SMX; fluoroquinolone for resistant organisms.

Discussion   Eighty percent of UTIs are caused by *E. coli*; *Staphylococcus saprophyticus* is the second most common cause. Other causes, in order of frequency, are *Proteus, Klebsiella, Enterobacter, Serratia, Pseudomonas,* and *Enterococcus*; *Chlamydia* and *Neisseria* are also causes of urethritis. Risk factors include female gender, sexual activity, pregnancy, obstruction, bladder dysfunction, vesicoureteral reflux, and catheterization.

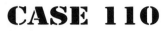

CASE 110

ID/CC	A 25-year-old **sexually active woman** presents with **burning during micturition** (DYSURIA), increased frequency and urgency of micturition, and low-grade fever.
HPI	She is otherwise in perfect health.
PE	VS: fever.
Labs	UA: abundant WBCs; mild proteinuria but no casts; staining of sediment reveals presence of gram-positive cocci. Urine culture isolates **coagulase-negative *Staphylococcus saprophyticus*.**
Treatment	Antibiotics (ampicillin, cotrimoxazole, or ciprofloxacin).
Discussion	Enterobacteriaceae such as *Escherichia coli, Klebsiella* species, and *Proteus* and *Pseudomonas* species are the most common organisms causing UTI. After *E. coli, Staphylococcus saprophyticus* is the most common cause of primary nonobstructive UTI in sexually active young women.

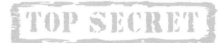

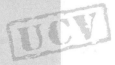

CASE 111

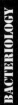

ID/CC   A 30-year-old male presents with sudden-onset fever, colicky **abdominal pain**, and **watery diarrhea**.

HPI   He had eaten **raw oysters** at a friend's party the day before (incubation period 4 hours to 4 days).

PE   VS: fever; tachycardia. PE: no dehydration; diffuse abdominal tenderness; increased bowel sounds.

Labs   *Vibrio parahaemolyticus* isolated from stool in a high-salt-content (halophilic vibrio) culture medium; PMNs in stool; **Kanagawa phenomenon** (beta-hemolysis on medium containing human blood; done as an indicator for pathogenicity) **positive**.

Treatment Fluid and electrolyte balance; antibiotics not required (since they do not shorten course of infection).

Discussion **Seafood** is the main source of the organism. After ingestion, *Vibrio parahaemolyticus* multiplies in the gut and produces a **diarrheal enterotoxin**.

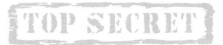

ID/CC   A 35-year-old male presents to the emergency room with high-grade fever, marked weakness, and a hemorrhagic **vesiculobullous skin eruption**.

HPI   He had just returned from deep-sea fishing in the Gulf of Mexico, where he had consumed large quantities of **seafood**. He has been diagnosed with **chronic liver disease** (due to hemochromatosis).

PE   VS: fever; hypotension; tachycardia. PE: icterus; vesiculobullous skin lesions seen on an otherwise-bronzed complexion.

Labs   Blood culture on **high-salt medium** (halophilic bacteria) reveals growth of *Vibrio vulnificus*; evidence of hemochromatosis (hyperglycemia, hyperbilirubinemia, increased serum iron).

Treatment   **Ceftazidime** and **doxycycline, ciprofloxacin**; supportive.

Discussion   Halophilic *Vibrio vulnificus* should be suspected and treated in any individual with chronic liver disease who presents with septicemia and skin lesions 1 to 3 days following seafood ingestion.

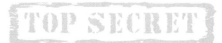

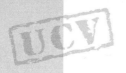

CASE 113

BACTERIOLOGY

ID/CC	A 56-year-old white male complains of **diarrhea** and bloating for **several months** along with ankle swelling.
HPI	He also complains of memory loss, fever, **arthritis** in the knees and hands, and **weight loss**.
PE	VS: fever. PE: thin, gaunt male; muscle wasting; swollen, tender right wrist and ankle; axillary and femoral lymphadenopathy; ecchymoses of chest and arms.
Labs	CBC/PBS: macrocytic, hypochromic anemia; hypoalbuminemia; **increased fecal fat** (steatorrhea). *Tropheryma whippelii* DNA detected on PCR.
Imaging	UGI/SBFT: nonspecific dilatation of small bowel.
Gross Pathology	Atrophy of intestinal mucosa; inflammatory infiltrate in synovia of joints.
Micro Pathology	Small bowel biopsy reveals **characteristic macrophages** containing bacilli with **PAS** reagent staining; characteristic gram-negative actinomycete bacilli in macrophages, PMNs, and epithelial cells of lamina propria; dilated lymphatics; flattening of intestinal villi.
Treatment	Bactrim (TMP-SMX), penicillin, or amoxicillin for several months until infection is eradicated.
Discussion	Caused by infection with *T. whippelii*; produces **malabsorption** of fat-soluble vitamins, protein, iron, folic acid, and vitamin B_{12}.

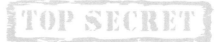

ID/CC   A 2-year-old female is brought to the emergency room because of **paroxysms** and multiple **coughs** in a single expiration, followed by a high-pitched **inspiratory whistle or whoop**.

HPI   For the past 2 weeks she has had a runny nose, low-grade fever, muscle pains, and headache. Her **immunization schedule is incomplete**.

PE   VS: fever. PE: child apprehensive and becomes cyanotic during cough paroxysm; thick green mucus expelled with cough; conjunctival injection.

Labs   CBC: **marked leukocytosis with lymphocytosis**. Diagnosis confirmed by culture on Bordet-Gengou medium.

Gross Pathology   Small conjunctival and brain hemorrhages may appear during paroxysms; bronchiectasis may also be a complication.

Micro Pathology   Signs of acute inflammation in upper respiratory tract mucosa, with erythema, petechiae, polymorphonuclear infiltrate, and necrosis.

Treatment   Largely supportive; **erythromycin** for treatment of patient and close contacts.

Discussion   A bacterial infection of the upper respiratory tract caused by *Bordetella pertussis*, a gram-negative coccobacillus, whooping cough is transmitted by droplets and comprises three stages: prodromal (catarrhal), paroxysmal (coughing), and convalescent. It is largely preventable with universally administered diphtheria toxoid, tetanus toxoid, and pertussis a cellular (DTP) vaccine. Pertussis toxin is a heat-labile exotoxin in which ADP ribosylates the inhibitory G protein, thus inactivating it and leading to constant activation of adenylate cyclase and increased cAMP. The remarkable lymphocytosis is due to pertussis toxin inhibiting chemokine receptors. As a result, lymphocytes are unable to leave the bloodstream.

ID/CC

A 10-year-old child who lives in tropical Africa presents with multiple papillomatous skin lesions and pain in both legs.

HPI

The first lesion had appeared on the leg as a small indurated papule that ulcerated into a granulomatous papilloma.

PE

Multiple papillomatous skin lesions seen, especially in intertriginous areas; lesions were painless and exuding a serous fluid; painful hyperkeratotic lesions seen on palms and soles; both tibia were tender to palpation.

Labs

Dark-field microscopic examination of exudate from lesions established the diagnosis by revealing organisms with the characteristic morphology and rotational motion of pathogenic treponemes; nontreponemal serologic tests (i.e., VDRL and RPR tests) and treponemal tests (i.e., FTA-ABS test) were positive.

Imaging

XR, legs: evidence of periostitis of the tibia.

Treatment

Long-acting intramuscular benzathine penicillin G is the treatment of choice.

Discussion

Yaws, the most common of the nonvenereal treponematoses, is a chronic infection of skin and bones caused by *Treponema pertenue*. Yaws occurs in tropical areas of Africa, Asia, and Central and South America; it is principally a disease of childhood, and initial infection occurs between 5 and 15 years of age. Transmission is by direct contact with infected skin lesions containing treponemes and is fostered by conditions of overcrowding and poor hygiene. The disease may occur in three stages: primary, secondary, and tertiary. Only lesions of primary and secondary yaws are infectious.

TOP SECRET

ID/CC   A 28-year-old female complains of **painful swelling of both knees** and **tender skin eruptions** on both shins.

HPI   For the past 2 weeks she has also had **watery diarrhea** that developed after she consumed some **raw pork**. She also complains of low-grade fever and mild abdominal pain.

PE   VS: low-grade fever; tachycardia. PE: mild dehydration; swollen and warm knee joints with painful restriction of all movements (ARTHRITIS); multiple **tender, erythematous plaques and nodules** (ERYTHEMA NODOSUM) seen over both shins.

Labs   CBC: leukocytosis. *Yersinia enterocolitica* isolated from stool; patient is **HLA-B27 positive**.

Micro Pathology   Oval ulcers with long axis in the direction of bowel flow, similar to ulcers caused by typhoid fever (intestinal tubercular ulcers are transverse).

Treatment   Supportive; antibiotics (aminoglycosides, fluoroquinolones) indicated in severe infections.

Discussion   *Yersinia enterocolitica* is an invasive gram-negative **intracellular pathogen** that causes **gastroenteritis**, most frequently involving the distal ileum and colon (enterotoxin mediated), **mesenteric adenitis** (due to necrotizing and suppurative gut lesions) and ileitis (**pseudoappendicitis**), and sepsis; infection may trigger a variety of **autoimmune phenomena**, including erythema nodosum, reactive arthritis, and possibly Graves' disease, especially in HLA-B27-positive individuals. Spread is by the fecal-oral route and occurs via contaminated milk products or water, swine, or household pet feces.

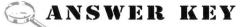
ANSWER KEY

1. Actinomycosis
2. Acute Bacterial Endocarditis
3. Acute Bronchiolitis
4. Acute Cystitis
5. Acute Rheumatic Fever
6. Acute Sinusitis
7. Anthrax
8. Aspiration Pneumonia with Lung Abscess
9. Atypical Mycobacterial Infection
10. Bacillus cereus Food Poisoning
11. Bacterial Vaginosis
12. Bartonellosis
13. Botulism
14. Brain Abscess
15. Breast Abscess
16. Brucellosis
17. Campylobacter Enteritis
18. Cat-Scratch Disease
19. Cellulitis
20. Chlamydia Pneumonia
21. Chlamydia trachomatis
22. Cholera
23. Chorioamnionitis
24. Diphtheria
25. Ehrlichiosis
26. Endemic Typhus
27. Epidemic Typhus
28. Epididymitis
29. Epiglottitis
30. Erysipelas
31. Erysipeloid
32. Fitz–Hugh–Curtis Syndrome
33. Gas Gangrene—Traumatic
34. Gastroenteritis—Staphylococcus aureus
35. Gonococcal Ophthalmia Neonatorum
36. Gonorrhea
37. Graft-Versus-Host Disease
38. Granuloma Inguinale
39. H. influenzae in a COPD Patient
40. Hemolytic-Uremic Syndrome (HUS)
41. Impetigo
42. Inclusion Conjunctivitis
43. Jarisch–Herxheimer Reaction
44. Legionella Pneumonia
45. Leprosy—Lepromatous

46. Leprosy—Tuberculoid
47. Leptospirosis (Weil's Disease)
48. Listeria Meningitis in the Newborn
49. Listeriosis
50. Lyme Disease
51. Lymphogranuloma Venereum
52. Meningitis—Bacterial (Adult)
53. Meningitis—Bacterial (Pediatric)
54. Meningitis—Tubercular
55. Meningococcemia
56. Mycoplasma Pneumonia
57. Necrotizing Enterocolitis
58. Necrotizing Fasciitis
59. Neutropenic Enterocolitis
60. Nocardiosis
61. Nosocomial Enterococcal Infection
62. Osteomyelitis
63. Otitis Externa
64. Otitis Media
65. Overwhelming Postsplenectomy Infections
66. Pasteurella multocida
67. Pelvic Inflammatory Disease
68. Pelvic Tuberculosis
69. Peptic Ulcer Disease (H. pylori)
70. Pharyngitis—Streptococcal
71. Plague
72. Pneumococcal Pneumonia
73. Pneumocystis carinii Pneumonia
74. Poststreptococcal Glomerulonephritis
75. Proctocolitis
76. Prostatitis—Acute
77. Prostatitis—Chronic
78. Prosthetic Valve Endocarditis
79. Psittacosis
80. Pyelonephritis—Acute
81. Pyogenic Liver Abscess
82. Q Fever
83. Rat Bite Fever
84. Relapsing Fever
85. Rocky Mountain Spotted Fever
86. Salmonella Food Poisoning
87. Salmonella Septicemia with Osteomyelitis
88. Scalded Skin Syndrome
89. Scarlet Fever

90. Septic Arthritis—Gonococcal
91. Shigellosis
92. Shock—Septic
93. Spontaneous Bacterial Peritonitis
94. Subacute Bacterial Endocarditis
95. Subdiaphragmatic Abscess
96. Syphilis—Congenital
97. Syphilis—Primary
98. Syphilis—Secondary
99. Syphilis—Tertiary (Tabes Dorsalis)
100. Tetanus
101. Tetanus Neonatorum
102. Toxic Shock Syndrome (TSS)
103. Traveler's Diarrhea

104. Tuberculosis—Miliary
105. Tuberculosis—Pulmonary
106. Tularemia
107. Typhoid Fever
108. Urethritis—Nongonococcal
109. Urinary Tract Infection (UTI)
110. UTI with Staphylococcus saprophyticus
111. Vibrio parahaemolyticus Food Poisoning
112. Vibrio vulnificus Food Poisoning
113. Whipple's Disease
114. Whooping Cough
115. Yaws
116. Yersinia Enterocolitis

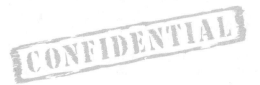

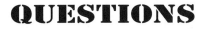

1. A few weeks after a camping trip on the Eastern seaboard of the U.S., an active 29-year-old female notices that she has been experiencing muscle aches and joint pains all over. Her friends comment that her smile seems a little "lopsided." On review of systems, she vaguely recalls a "weird rash" that went away. The best explanation for her complaints is:

   A: Chagas' disease
   B: Gonorrhea
   C: Lyme disease
   D: Rocky Mountain spotted fever
   E: Sleeping sickness

2. A 32-year-old male presents to your office after a 5-day vacation in Myrtle Beach, South Carolina. He complains of a circular red, itchy patch of skin on his right forearm. You examined the area under a Wood's lamp and discover it fluoresces green. This tells you:

   A: Further examination of this area is warranted to narrow down the fungal species infecting the individual.
   B: This is a dermatophyte infection of the *Epidermophyton* species.
   C: This is a dermatophyte infection of the *Microsporum* species.
   D: This is a dermatophyte infection of the *Trichophyton* species.
   E: This is an erythema migrans rash of Lyme disease.

3. You're working in the family practice clinic and a breast feeding woman who is 22 years old presents with a painful mass in the inferior portion of her left breast. Your exam reveals a fluctuant mass that is tender and warm. You can expect green tinted breast milk on exam. You tell her which of the following?

   A: We will set you up with a surgeon who will take a small needle biopsy just to make sure no cancer is present.
   B: Encourage frequent breast feeding and give her an antibiotic.
   C: Tell her to stop nursing all together and let the infection heal.
   D: We will set you up for a mammogram today.
   E: We will call the surgeon and see if an excisional biopsy can be performed today, we will also set you up with an oncology appointment.

4. A previously healthy 3-month-old boy is brought to the hospital with a high fever, decreased interest in breast feeding and inconsolable crying. As part of the workup, the patient has a lumbar puncture, which reveals bacterial meningitis. The most likely causes of bacterial meningitis in newborns are:

   A: Group B Streptococci, *E. coli*, and *Listeria*
   B: *Listeria* and *E. coli*
   C: *N. meningitidis* and *H. influenza* B
   D: *S. pneumonia* and gram-negative rods
   E: *Staphyococcus aureus* and *Klebsiella pneumonia*

5. A 37-year-old AIDS patient visits a relative in Arizona. During his visit he develops meningeal symptoms and nuchal rigidity. After a spinal tap and analysis of the spinal fluid, you diagnose the patient with fungal meningitis. The most likely cause of fungal meningitis in this patient is:

   A: Blastomycosis
   B. *Candida*
   C: Coccidioidomycosis
   D: Histoplasmosis
   E: Paracoccidioidomycosis

6. A college rugby player comes to student health for a hot inflamed knee. It has been this way for almost 5 days since a big game this past weekend. He does not remember injuring it, nor can you find any evidence of a scrape. The left knee has the following qualities: calor, dolor, rubor. He is limited to his range of motion and cannot walk due to the pain. You aspirate the knee and Gram stain it yourself. Your findings are as follows: bean-shaped gram-negative diplococci. You infer than your history should have included which of the following?

   A: Eye exam
   B: History of IV drug use
   C: History of passing out
   D: History of trauma within the past year
   E: Sexual history

7. A patient comes into your office for her prenatal visit. She is currently 4 weeks pregnant and has no complaints. She casually mentions that she is thinking about adopting a kitten for her 5-year-old son so that he won't be jealous when the baby comes. This will be the first time that she has owned a kitten. You are most concerned about what infection?

   A: Cat scratch fever
   B: CMV
   C: *Francisella*
   D: Rubella
   E: Toxoplasmosis

8. A 62-year-old woman has been admitted several times in the past few months for fever workup. She lives on a cattle farm in the Midwestern U.S. and has, up to this past year, been in excellent health. She tells the team that she had an episode several months ago when she experienced muscle aches, night sweats, a profound headache, and cough. Her husband says that her eyeballs turned yellow. On this present admission, a new heart murmur is noted. Blood cultures for endocarditis have returned negative results. The most likely organism causing her fever is:

   A: *Coxiella burnetii*
   B: *Leishmania donovani*

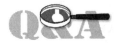

C: *Shigella flexneri*
D: *Streptococcus pneumoniae*
E: *Treponema pallidum*

9. A 29-year-old male returns from a 2-day trip to Mexico with frequent loose stools that do not contain blood. You diagnose the patient with traveler's diarrhea. Of the following organisms, which is most likely to cause non-bloody, watery diarrhea?

    A: *Campylobacter jejuni*
    B: *Entamoeba histolytica*
    C: Enterotoxigenc *E. coli*
    D: *Salmonella*
    E: *Shigella*

10. A 30-year-old male comes into your clinic complaining of a maculopapular rash on his palms and soles that first appeared 2 weeks ago. He also complains of general malaise and poor appetite within the past few weeks. Upon further questioning, he states that he had a painless ulcer on the shaft of his penis which healed spontaneously after a month. He currently has unprotected sex with several female partners, but has never been tested for any STD. What is the most likely diagnosis?

    A: Syphilis
    B: Herpes virus
    C: Rocky mountain spotted fever
    D: Gonorrhea
    E: *Chlamydia*

11. A 6-year-old boy with sickle cell anemia comes into the hospital complaining of knee pain. On exam, you find a tender swollen knee joint without signs of draining from the skin. An x-ray of the knee shows osteomyelitis. Abdominal films confirm that the patient does not have a spleen. What is the most likely organism?

    A: *Neisseria gonorrhoeae*
    B: *Pseudomonas aeruginosa*
    C: *Salmonella*
    D: *Staph epidermidis*
    E: Tuberculosis

12. You just got results from the micro lab about the *Staphylococcus* species growing in your patient's culture. It's just before rounds and you were just able to get the following information: + beta hemolysis, + catalase, + coagulase, protein A present, biotin not required for growth. You do not want to look ignorant on round and tell the attending that according to the microlab that *Staph* species is:

A: *Aureus*
B: *Epidermidis*
C: *Pyogenes*
D: *Saprophyticus*

13. A 45-year-old white male presents with left lower leg pain. Exam reveals a well-demarcated region that is hot, erythematous, swollen, and exquisitely tender. Frank pus is noted and collected. Culture on sheep's blood agar produces a clear zone around colonies. You suspect Group A streptococcus. What lab test will help confirm this diagnosis?

A: CAMP test
B: Grows in hypertonic NaCl
C: Hydrolyze esculin in bile
D: Hydrolyze hippurate
E: Inhibition by bacitracin
F: Inhibited by optochin

14. A 34-year-old HIV patient is admitted for fever of unknown origin and is noted to have a new heart murmur. Physical findings include splinter hemorrhages, Janeway lesions, and focal neurological findings. Blood cultures are obtained but no organisms are found. The most likely organism causing this patient's endocarditis is:

A: *N. gonorrhoeae*
B: *S. aureus*
C: *Eikenella*
D: *S. pneumoniae*
E: *T. cruzi*

15. A 24-year-old female with a past medical history of recurrent urinary tract infections presents to your office with suprapubic pain, fever, and urinary urgency and frequency. On urinalysis you find that the urine has an alkaline pH, increased leukocyte esterase, and increased nitrate. A likely cause of the patient's infection is:

A: *E. coli*
B: *Proteus mirabilis*
C: *Pseudomonas*
D: *Staphylococcus saphrophyticus*
E: *Streptococcus pneumonia*

16. A 26-year-old white female presents to the outpatient clinic complaining of an expanding rash. Social history is significant for recent backpacking on the Appalachian Trail in New England. The rash is localized to her upper back, and appears erythematous and circular with central clearing. The patient recalls no tick bite. Doxycycline is initiated. What is the make-up of the vaccine recommended in endemic areas?

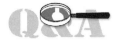

A: Bacillus Calmette-Guérin (BCG)
B: Live, attenuated bacterium (acid-fast negative)
C: Outer surface protein
D: Polysaccharide conjugated to toxoid
E: Toxoid
F: Vi capsular polysaccharide

17. A 20-year-old college woman comes into the ED with complaints of severe throbbing headache, fever, neck stiffness, nausea, vomiting, and photophobia that started several hours ago. She also noticed a rash that had developed on her extremities. She took Tylenol and Benadryl to help her sleep, but the pain is unbearable. You decide to do a lumbar puncture after confirming that she does not have increased intracranial pressure. Her CSF revealed an increase in WBC with predominant neutrophils, decreased glucose, and gram negative diplococci. What organism is the cause of her meningitis?

    A: Group B streptococcus
    B: *Haemophilus influenzae*
    C: *Listeria monocytogenes*
    D: *Streptococcus pneumoniae*
    E: *Neisseria meningitidis*

18. A family of four comes into the ER complaining of abdominal pain, diarrhea, and nausea and vomiting after attending a picnic on a hot summer day. They recall eating well cooked hamburgers, potato salad, watermelon, and lemonade. What is the most likely organism responsible for the food poisoning?

    A: *Bacillus cereus*
    B: *Clostridium botulinum*
    C: *Staph aureus*
    D: *E. coli*
    E: *Salmonella*

19. You are asked by an attending to evaluate a 59-year-old male who was first infected with tuberculosis 30 years ago. He recently had a kidney transplant for which he takes immunosuppressive drugs. The attending suspects that he has symptoms of Pott's disease. What area of the body does this involve?

    A: CNS
    B: Kidneys
    C: Lungs
    D: Testicles
    E: Vertebrae

20. A 22-year-old female presents to the gynecologist with complaints of pain and frequency with urination for 2 days. Urine analysis shows a urine pH of

8 (elevated from normal). Urine cultures show colonies swarming to cover the entire plate. What is the most likely organism causing this UTI?

A: *E. coli*
B: *Pseudomonas*
C: *Proteus mirabilis*
D: *Serratia*
E: *Staph saprophyticus*

ANSWERS

1.   C

A: Chagas' disease [Incorrect] This is caused by *Trypanosoma cruzi*. It is spread by reduviid insects, typically in South America. A nodule, or chagoma, forms at the site of insect bite. Later complications include megacolon, megaesophagus, and cardiac abnormalities (conduction block).

B: Gonorrhea [Incorrect] While disseminated gonorrhea can cause joint pains, this organism is better known for monoarticular manifestations. In addition, it is not associated with cranial nerve palsies.

C: Lyme disease [Correct] *Borrelia burgdorferi* is a tick-borne spirochete that is classically associated with erythema chronicum migrans, often missed by patients. This patient manifested other signs, such as her malaise and arthralgias. Her facial droop is also a classic finding for Lyme disease. A tetracycline will be helpful in eradicating the disease.

D: Rocky Mountain spotted fever [Incorrect] This is caused by a tick-borne *Rickettsia* (*R. rickettsii*). It presents with headache, fever, and a generalized skin rash (palms and soles first).

E: Sleeping sickness [Incorrect] Also known as African trypanosomiasis, sleeping sickness is not found on the Eastern seaboard of the U.S. Fever, lymphadenopathy, joint pains, and CNS changes are characteristic.

2.   C

A: Further examination of this area is warranted to narrow down the fungal species infecting the individual. [Incorrect] Of the species causing dermatophyte infections only *Microsporum* will fluoresce under a Wood's lamp.

B: This is a dermatophyte infection of the *Epidermophyton* species. [Incorrect] *Epidermophyton* species do not fluoresce under a Wood's lamp. *E. floccosum* infects skin and nails but not hair.

C: This is a dermatophyte infection of the *Microsporum* species. [Correct] Certain *Microsporum* species, when hairs are involved, will fluoresce under a Wood's lamp. *Microsporum* species only infect hair and skin.

D: This is a dermatophyte infection of the *Trichophyton* species. [Incorrect] Lyme disease is caused by *Borrelia burgdorferi*, which is transmitted by a tick bite.

E: This is an erythema migrans rash of Lyme disease. [Incorrect] The erythema migrans rash, usually described as a "bulls-eye" rash does not fluoresce under a Wood's lamp. It is the hallmark rash of Lyme disease. Lyme disease is caused by *Borrelia bergdorferi*, which is transmitted by a tick bite.

3. B

    A: We will set you up with a surgeon who will take a small needle biopsy just to make sure no cancer is present. [Incorrect]

    B: Encourage frequent breast feeding and give her an antibiotic. [Correct] Frequent breast feeding has been shown to shorten the clinical course of mastitis along with abx treatment. The organisms will be killed in the infant's stomach and the antibiotic must be safe for infants.

    C: Tell her to stop nursing all together and let the infection heal. [Incorrect] This will likely lengthen the clinical course and possibly cause abscess.

    D: We will set you up for a mammogram today. [Incorrect] There is no current indication for mammogram and due to the density of the breast tissue the study would not find many small cancers if they existed.

    E: We will call the surgeon and see if an excisional biopsy can be performed today, we will also set you up with an oncology appointment. [Incorrect]

4. A

    A: Group B streptococci, *E. coli*, and *Listeria*. [Correct] Group B streptococci, *E. coli*, and *Listeria* are the common causes of meningitis in newborns.

    B: *Listeria* and *E. coli*. [Incorrect] While *Listeria* and *E. coli* are common causes of meningitis in the newborn, answer A is correct because it includes Group B streptococci, a common cause of meningitis in newborns.

    C: *N. meningitidis* and *H. influenza* B. [Incorrect] *N. meningitidis* and *H. influenza* B are common causes of meningitis in children, but not newborns. The incidence of *H. influenza* B is decreasing due to the widespread use of the prevnar vaccine against *H. influenza* B.

    D: *S. pneumonia* and gram-negative rods. [Incorrect] *S. pneumonia* is an uncommon cause of meningitis in newborns, but it is a common cause of meningitis in children and adults. Gram-negative rods is a common cause of meningitis in the elderly.

    E: *Staphylococcus aureus* and *Klebsiella pneumonia*. [Incorrect] *Staphlococcus aureus* and *Klebsiella pneumonia* are rare causes of meningitis.

5. C

    A: Blastomycosis. [Incorrect] Blastomycosis is endemic in the Ohio, Mississippi, and St. Lawrence River valleys and it is more likely to cause pulmonary disease rather than meningitis.

    B: *Candida*. [Incorrect] While *Candida* can cause meningitis, coccidioidomycosis is more likely to cause meningitis than *Candida*.

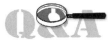

C: Coccidioidomycosis. [Correct] Coccidioidomycosis is endemic in the southwestern U.S. and California. It is known to cause fungal meningitis in immunocompromised patients. It can be treated with fluconazole.

D: Histoplasmosis. [Incorrect] Histoplasmosis is a fungus that is endemic in the Mississippi and Ohio River valleys. Histoplasmosis is more likely to cause pulmonary disease than to cause meningitis.

E: Paracoccidioidomycosis. [Incorrect] Paracoccidioidomycosis is endemic in rural South America. Paracoccidioidomycosis usually causes pulmonary disease, but disseminated disease may occur.

6. E

A: Eye exam [Incorrect] The eye exam would be noncontributory in this case.

B: History of IV drug use [Incorrect] While this may have been important if we had found evidence of staphylococcus or less likely *Strep*, with the following Gram stain it is not that important.

C: History of passing out [Incorrect] The history of passing out would not help us diagnose this acute illness, but would require workup and listening for aortic stenosis.

D: History of trauma within the past year [Incorrect] There are known latent joint infections of healthy persons.

E: Sexual history [Correct] This is the classical description of gonococcal arthritis, a sexual history is always important; specifically in young people with a septic joint. This requires immediate therapy, commonly with IV ceftriaxone.

7. E

A: Cat scratch fever [Incorrect] Patients can become infected with *Bartonella henselae* following a cat bite or scratch. Symptoms include regional lymphadenopathy, low grade fever, and general malaise, but patients usually recover within a few months without complications.

B: CMV [Incorrect] Infected women are often asymptomatic. The rate of transmission is highest with primary infections. Most infants affected with CMV will have hearing loss. Only a small percentage of infants have acute symptoms consisting of chorioretinitis and pneumonitis.

C: *Francisella* [Incorrect] *Francisella tularensis* is usually acquired from handling infected rabbits and from tick or deerfly bites. It is very virulent and can cause severe systemic infections. It is unlikely that a kitten from a pet shop or animal shelter will be infected with these bacteria.

D: Rubella [Incorrect] The rubella vaccine is typically given in childhood (MMR vaccine), but pregnant women should be tested for antibody titers. The rubella vaccine is live attenuated and therefore should not be given to pregnant women. Symptoms of infection include an upper respiratory infection, arthritis, and facial rash. Rate of fetal transmission is very high during the first trimester. Congenital anomalies include mental retardation, retinopathy, "blueberry muffin" rash, and cardiac defects.

E: Toxoplasmosis [Correct] *Toxoplasma gondii* is a parasite found in cat feces and raw meat. Primary infection with *T. gondii* during pregnancy increases the risk of congenital toxoplasmosis which includes jaundice, hydrocephalus, chorioretinitis, and intracranial calcifications. This infection can then lead to deafness, blindness, mental retardation, and seizures. You should advise your patient to wait until she has delivered to adopt the kitten. Pregnant women who were previously infected with *T. gondii* are not at risk of transmitting it to their fetuses.

8. A

A: *Coxiella burnetii* [Correct] This *Rickettsia* is responsible for Q fever, which is the cause of this patient's fever of unknown origin. The organism is found in cattle and sheep (especially in products of conception) and is highly resistant to drying. It is usually inhaled from infected dust. Q fever presents with fever, atypical pneumonia, myalgia, night sweats, profound headache, and hepatitis. When untreated, chronic Q fever can lead to endocarditis.

B: *Leishmania donovani* [Incorrect] This protozoa causes visceral leishmaniasis, or kala-azar, which presents as hyperpigmentation, night sweats, fevers, splenomegaly, and weight loss. It occurs in Africa, the Middle East, the Mediterranean, and India.

C: *Shigella flexneri* [Incorrect] This gram negative bacteria causes diarrhea.

D: *Streptococcus pneumoniae* [Incorrect] This gram positive organism causes pneumonia.

E: *Treponema pallidum* [Incorrect] The patient's presentation is not consistent with syphilis.

9. C

A: *Campylobacter jejuni.* [Incorrect] *Campylobacter jejuni* is a common cause of bloody diarrhea. *Campylobacter jejuni* is also one of the agents associated with Guillain-Barré disease.

B: *Entamoeba histolytica.* [Incorrect] *Entamoeba histolytica* is a protozoa that causes bloody diarrhea.

C: Enterotoxigenic *E. coli.* [Correct] Enterotoxigenic *E. coli* is the most common causative agent in traveler's diarrhea and causes a non-bloody watery diarrhea.

D: *Salmonella.* [Incorrect] *Salmonella* causes bloody diarrhea.

E: *Shigella.* [Incorrect] *Shigella* commonly causes bloody diarrhea.

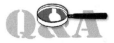

10. A

A: Syphilis [Correct] This patient presents with secondary syphilis, which develops after the chancre heals. If untreated, the symptoms will heal as the disease enters the latent period, during which time, the disease can still be transmitted to his sexual partners. Given the high clinical suspicion, it is best to confirm the diagnosis with the fluorescent treponemal antibody absorption test (FTA-ABS). Penicillin G is the treatment of choice, with doxycycline or tetracycline given to patients with penicillin allergies.

B: Herpes virus [Incorrect] Patients with HSV present with clear vesicles that can form painful ulcers after rupturing. The diagnostic test is a Tzanck smear from a culture of the ulcer base which will show multinucleated giant cells. Treatment with acyclovir can shorten the period of outbreaks, but is not curative.

C: Rocky Mountain spotted fever [Incorrect] Although RMSF can also present with a rash that appears on the soles, palms, wrists, and ankles, patients usually also complain of fever, conjunctival injection, and severe headaches. Given his history of a healed painless ulcer and unprotected sex, syphilis is the more likely diagnosis.

D: Gonorrhea [Incorrect] Gonorrhea can present as cervicitis or urethritis with purulent discharge and dysuria in females and is often asymptomatic in males. Culture of the discharge will show gram-negative intracellular diplococci. Treat with 3rd generation cephalosporins.

E: *Chlamydia* [Incorrect] 50% of patients with gonorrhea will be co-infected with *Chlamydia*. It is often asymptomatic, but can present as urethritis or cervicitis with mucopurulent discharge in females and mucopurulent urethral discharge in males. DNA probes and immunofluorescence studies are used to confirm the diagnosis. Treat with doxycycline or azithromycin.

11. C

A: *Neisseria gonorrhoeae* [Incorrect] This is a leading cause of septic arthritis in sexually active patients. Most patients will have signs of dissemination such as petechial rash or necrosis of the skin.

B: *Pseudomonas aeruginosa* [Incorrect] This is most often seen in diabetic or immunocompromised patients. If it infects a skin wound, it will give off a characteristic almond scent.

C: *Salmonella* [Correct] Sickle cell patients usually infarct their spleens around the age of 6. They are more vulnerable to encapsulated organisms such as salmonella. HOWEVER, *S. aureus* is the most common cause of osteomyelitis, even in sickle cell patients. If it was given in the choices, *S. aureus* would have been the correct answer.

D: *Staph epidermidis* [Incorrect] This infection is mostly often seen after joint surgery such as knee replacement. It is due to direct inoculation of the skin flora into the bone.

E: Tuberculosis [Incorrect] Although TB can spread to the bones, it most likely involves the vertebral column. TB of the spine occurs with reactivated TB or in someone who has had TB for many years. In this young patient, TB of the bones is very unlikely.

12. A

A: *Areus* [Correct]

B: *Epiderims* [Incorrect] Variable hemolysis, + catalase, − coagulase, Protein A absent, biotin required for growth.

C: *Pyogenes* [Incorrect] Beta hemolysis, − catalase, neg coagulase, absent Protein A, biotin not required for growth.

D: *Saprophyticus* [Incorrect] Variable hemolysis, positive catalase, neg coagulase absent protein A, biotin not required for growth.

13. E

A: CAMP test. [Incorrect] Group B streptococcus, or *Streptococcus agalactiae*, is found in the female genital tract, and often causes neonatal meningitis and sepsis. Group B streptococcus is also bacitracin resistant, and demonstrates beta-hemolysis on sheep's blood agar.

B: Grows in hypertonic NaCl. [Incorrect] Enterococci, a division of Group D streptococcus, are resistant to conditions in the harsh environment of the intestines. Enterococci often cause urinary tract infections.

C: Hydrolyze esculin in bile. [Incorrect] Group D streptococci are potential agents for endocarditis. These bacteria demonstrate alpha-hemolysis on sheep's blood agar, leaving a green halo rather than clearing.

D: Hydrolyze hippurate. [Incorrect] *Streptococcus agalactiae* can hydrolyze hippurate as a unique characteristic.

E: Inhibition by bacitracin. [Correct] Bacitracin sensitivity is diagnostic of *Streptococcus pyogenes*, or Group A hemolytic streptococcus. This bacterium is responsible for many cases of pharyngitis, cellulites, scarlet fever, and streptococcal toxic shock syndrome. The clear zone of hemolysis is consistent with beta-hemolysis, another characteristic of *Streptococcus pyogenes*.

F: Inhibited by optochin. [Incorrect] *Streptococcus pneumoniae*, gram positive diplococci, are inhibited by optochin. This bacterium is responsible for pneumonia characterized by rusty, brown sputum, and is a major agent in upper respiratory infections. A 23-valent polysaccharide vaccine is used for prophylaxis.

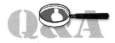

14. C

A: *N. gonorrhoeae* [Incorrect] Routine blood cultures would have detected this organism.

B: *S. aureus* [Incorrect] Routine blood cultures would have detected this organism.

C: *Eikenella* [Correct] Because the blood cultures were negative, it is likely that this patient has contracted a culture-negative endocarditis, which is associated with the HACEK organisms (*Hemophilus parainfluenzae, Actinobacillus, Cardiobacterium, Eikenella, Kingella*).

D: *S. pneumoniae* [Incorrect] Routine blood cultures would have detected this organism.

E: *T. cruzi* [Incorrect] The causative agent for Chagas' disease, trypanosomiasis typically presents as a conduction abnormality in the right bundle branch.

15. B

A: *E. coli.* [Incorrect] While *E. coli* causes 50–80% of urinary tract infections in non-hospitalized patients, it is not a urease splitting organism. The high pH of the urine suggests that a urease splitting organism is the cause of the infection.

B: *Proteus mirabalis.* [Correct] Patients with urinary tract infections due to *Proteus* or other urease splitting organisms will have urine with an alkaline pH. Theses patients also have an increased incidence of struvite kidney stones.

C: *Pseudomonas.* [Incorrect] *Pseudomonas* is a common cause of noso-comial urinary tract infections, but not community acquired urinary tract infections. *Pseudomonas* is not a urease splitting organism.

D: *Staphylococcus saprophyticus.* [Incorrect] *Staphylococcus saprophyticus* causes 10–30% of urinary tract infections in ambulatory patients and it is not a urease splitting organism.

E: *Streptococcus pneumonia.* [Incorrect] *Streptococcus pneumonia* is not a known cause of urinary tract infections.

16. C

A: Bacillus Calmette-Guérin (BCG). [Incorrect] This live strain of *Mycobacterium bovis* is used to generate partial immunity to *Mycobacterium tuberculosis*. BCG vaccine is not used in the United States due to the loss of utility of the tuberculin skin test. Any Mycobacterium exposure can induce a positive PPD response. Only BCG and the *Francisella tularensis* vaccines are live, attenuated bacterial vaccines.

B: Live, attenuated bacterium (acid-fast negative). [Incorrect] People with exposure to wild animals are encouraged to receive *Francisella tularensis* vaccination. Tularemia is spread most often by ticks from rabbit reservoir. Only BCG and the *Francisella tularensis* vaccines are live, attenuated bacterial vaccines.

C: Outer surface protein. [Correct] *Borrelia burgdorferi*, the infectious agent in Lyme disease, is spread by tick bite. Half of patients with Lyme disease cannot recount a tick bite. The recommended vaccine consists of recombinant outer surface protein (OspA), administered in three doses.

D: Polysaccharide conjugated to toxoid. [Incorrect] *Haemophilus influenzae* historically was a primary cause of meningitis, epiglottitis, and upper respiratory tract infections in children. The effective vaccine, which consists of *Haemophilus influenzae* capsular polysaccharide conjugated to diphtheria toxoid or another toxoid, has dramatically reduced the impact of *Haemophilus influenzae*.

E: Toxoid. [Incorrect] Tetanus, pertussis, and diphtheria vaccines include toxoids. A toxoid is a toxin that retains antigenicity with minimal or no toxic effects. Toxoids may be produced by treating the toxin with formaldehyde or by genetically altering the protein.

F: Vi capsular polysaccharide. [Incorrect] *Samonella typhi* vaccine contains Vi capsular polysaccharide, but offers little protection. Only 50–75% of patients may receive protective benefits from the typhoid vaccine.

17. E

A: Group B streptococcus [Incorrect] This is usually seen in neonates. GBS appears as gram positive lancets in chains. It is important to remember that neonates with meningitis will show nonspecific signs such as fever, vomiting, poor feeding, and irritability.

B: *Haemophilus influenzae* [Incorrect] This is rare in the U.S. because routine vaccinations are given early in life. However, when it does occur, it is often in young children. *H. influenzae* appears as gram negative rods.

C: *Listeria monocytogenes* [Incorrect] This is most often seen in neonates, immunosuppressed people, and pregnant women. *L. monocytogenes* appears as gram positive motile rods.

D: *Streptococcus pneumoniae* [Incorrect] Although this is a common cause of meningitis in the adult population, *S. pneumoniae* appears as lancet shaped gram-positive diplococci.

E: *Neisseria meningitidis* [Correct] *N. meningitidis* is spread by respiratory transmission and is the most common cause of meningitis in people who reside in close quarters, such as army recruits or college students who live in dorms. The petechial rash is diagnostic for *N. meningitidis* infection. Prompt treatment with high dose IV antibiotics is essential in decreasing the risk of neurologic sequelae.

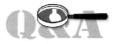

18. C

A: *Bacillus cereus* [Incorrect] *B. cereus* is usually found in reheated rice. Spores are deposited on food and can survive the initial cooking process. They can only be killed with high temperatures or refrigeration.

B: *Clostridium botulinum* [Incorrect] *C. botulinum* spores are usually found in home canned foods. They cause descending paralysis in adults. They can also be found in honey, and if given to babies, will cause a flaccid paralysis.

C: *Staph aureus* [Correct] Pre-formed toxins are usually found in mayonnaise that has not been properly refrigerated and cause rapid development of food poisoning. Always think of *S. aureus* if someone mentions that they just came back from a picnic and had eaten foods containing mayonnaise such as potato salad.

D: *E. coli* [Incorrect] *E. coli* 0157:H7 is usually found in undercooked foods. Since the family states that the hamburgers were well cooked, this is less likely to be the culprit.

E: *Salmonella* [Incorrect] Food poisoning from salmonella usually occurs after eating improperly cooked poultry, meat, or eggs.

19. E

A: CNS [Incorrect] TB can lead to granuloma formation in the brain and cause meningitis.

B: Kidneys [Incorrect] Spread to the kidneys is usually hematogenous. Patients present with nonspecific urinary tract infections. The kidneys can become atrophic, scarred, densely calcified, and non-functioning if not appropriately treated.

C: Lungs [Incorrect] If the patient's primary TB is reactivated, a caseating cavitary lesion is seen on chest x-ray and the patient will complain of hemoptysis or coughing up blood.

D: Testicles [Incorrect] TB that has spread to the genitals can lead to infertility. Nodular beading of the vas is a characteristic physical finding. Orchitis and testicular swelling can occur.

E: Vertebrae [Correct] Immunosuppressed patients are more likely to manifest complications of TB infection. Pott's disease is extrapulmonary spread of TB to the vertebrae. This can lead to softening and collapse of the spinal column, causing a hunchback deformity.

20. C

A: *E. coli* [Incorrect] *E. coli* is a common cause of UTI as it is abundant in feces. Women who wipe in an anal to vaginal direction can spread the organism to the vaginal area. Gram stains and culture will show gram-negative rods.

B: *Pseudomonas* [Incorrect] This is usually a nosocomial or hospital acquired cause of UTI. It will produce a big-green pigment on urine culture.

C: *Proteus mirabilis* [Correct] If a patient with a UTI has an alkaline pH on the urine analysis, think *Proteus*. These organisms are able to split urea into ammonia and CO_2. They are very motile. On a plate smear, they will form a confluence of colonies that rapidly grow to cover the entire plate.

D: *Serratia* [Incorrect] *Serratia* is known to produce a red pigment on urine cultures. In infected babies, it causes the red diaper finding.

E: *Staph saprophyticus* [Incorrect] Although this is the leading cause of UTI in the community and in sexually active females, it does not cause alkaline urine. Gram stains and urine cultures will show gram-positive cocci in clusters.